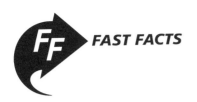

MW00845920

Fast Facts: Immuno-Oncology

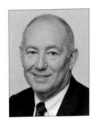

Stephen Clarke OAM MBBS PhD MD FRACP FAChPM
Director, Area Cancer Services
Northern Sydney Local Health District
Professor of Medicine, University of Sydney
Royal North Shore Hospital
New South Wales, Australia

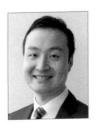

Bob T Li MD MPH MBBS FRACP
Attending Medical Oncologist
Thoracic Oncology and Early Drug Development Service
Memorial Sloan Kettering Cancer Center
New York, USA

Declaration of Independence
This book is as balanced and as practical as we can make it.
Ideas for improvement are always welcome: feedback@fastfacts.com

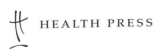
HEALTH PRESS

Fast Facts: Immuno-Oncology
First published November 2017

Health Press Limited, Elizabeth House, Queen Street, Abingdon,
Oxford OX14 3LN, UK
Tel: +44 (0)1235 523233

Book orders can be placed by telephone or via the website.
For regional distributors or to order via the website, please go to:
fastfacts.com
For telephone orders, please call +44 (0)1752 202301

Fast Facts is a trademark of Health Press Limited.

The publisher and the authors have made every effort to ensure
the accuracy of this book, but cannot accept responsibility for any
errors or omissions.

For all drugs, please consult the product labeling approved in your
country for prescribing information.

A CIP record for this title is available from the British Library.

ISBN 978-1-910797-70-9

Clarke S (Stephen)
Fast Facts: Immuno-Oncology/
Stephen Clarke, Bob T Li

Cover image is a conceptual illustration of T cells attacking
cancer cells marked by monoclonal antibodies.
Evan Oto/Science Photo Library.

Medical illustrations by Graeme Chambers.
Typesetting by Thomas Bohm, User Design, Illustration
and Typesetting, UK.
Printed in the UK with Xpedient Print.

Glossary

Abscopal response: a response to radiotherapy that is achieved at sites distant from the treatment site

ACT: adoptive cell transfer – a form of cell-based cancer immunotherapy in which circulating or tumor-infiltrating lymphocytes are collected from the patient, modified ex vivo as necessary to attack the patient's specific neoantigens, and reinfused into the patient

Adaptive (acquired) immunity: immunity conferred by the formation of antibodies following exposure to foreign material (antigens)

ADCC: antibody-dependent cell-mediated cytotoxicity – a cell-mediated immune mechanism in which an effector cell of the immune system lyses a target cell, the surface antigens of which have been bound by specific antibodies

Adjuvant: a compound that augments the immune response to an antigen

Anergy: a state of non-activity induced in maturing lymphocytes following exposure to self-antigens

Antigen: a substance capable of triggering an immune response by binding to an antibody

APC: antigen-presenting cell

Apoptosis: programmed cell death

BCG: Bacillus Calmette–Guérin – an adjuvant used to stimulate an immune response in the production of vaccines

BCR: B cell receptor

BiTE®: bispecific T-cell engager – a chimeric protein consisting of two single-chain variable fragments from separate monoclonal antibodies, one targeting a tumor-associated antigen, and the other targeting a T-cell surface antigen

CAR-T: chimeric antigen receptor-expressing T cell – a lymphocyte that has been genetically modified to express a transmembrane protein consisting of the tumor-associated antigen-binding domain of an antibody linked to one or more immunostimulatory domains

CCL22: a chemokine that promotes trafficking of regulatory T cells to tumor sites

CD22: a non-specific receptor inhibitor that reduces the activation of B cell receptors

CEACAM1: carcinoembryonic antigen-related cell adhesion molecule 1 – an adhesion molecule that is expressed by natural killer cells and T lymphocytes, and is over-expressed in most melanomas

Cellular (cell-mediated) immunity: acquired immune responses mediated by T lymphocytes

Chemokine: a cytokine that promotes recruitment of inflammatory or immune cells to sites of injury or infection

Complement: a cascade of plasma proteins that facilitates (or 'complements') the ability of antibodies to eliminate pathogens

CRS: cytokine release syndrome

CSC: cancer stem cell

CTLA-4: cytotoxic T-lymphocyte-associated protein 4 – a protein that plays a key role in deactivated cytotoxic CD8+ T cells through binding to CD80 (B7-1) on antigen-presenting cells

Cytokines: chemical mediators produced by inflammatory cells at sites of infection or injury, which trigger further recruitment of inflammatory cells

Cytotoxic (CD8+) T cells: a class of T cells (also known as killer T cells) that induce the death of damaged cells, such as cells infected with viruses or other pathogens

DAMP: damage-associated molecular pattern – a molecule produced in response to tissue damage that is recognized by immune cells expressing pattern recognition receptors

Dendritome: a fusion between a dendritic cell and an inactivated cancer cell, which is intended to prime immune responses directed against tumor-associated antigens

EGFR: epidermal growth factor receptor

Epitope spreading: the acquired ability of an immunotherapy directed against a specific antigen to react to multiple antigens

GM-CSF: granulocyte macrophage colony-stimulating factor

HMGB1: high mobility group box 1 – a damage-associated molecular pattern released following immunogenic cell death

Humoral immunity: acquired immune responses mediated by B lymphocytes

ICD: immunogenic cell death – a form of apoptosis triggered by certain forms of chemotherapy and radiotherapy

IDO: indoleamine 2,3-dioxygenase – an enzyme that depletes intracellular supplies of tryptophan, which is needed for T-cell proliferation

IFN: interferon

IL: interleukin

IMiD: immunomodulatory drug

Immune checkpoints: receptor-ligand systems that, when activated, downregulate immune responses to prevent autoimmunity, minimize damage to healthy tissue during an immune response, or both

Immune tolerance: a state in which the immune system is unresponsive to a stimulus that would normally provoke an immune response

Immunogenicity: the ability (e.g. of a cancer cell) to trigger an immune response

Innate immunity: immunity conferred by mechanisms present throughout life

irRC: immune-related response criteria

LPS: lipopolysaccharide – an adjuvant used to stimulate an immune response in the production of vaccines

mAb: monoclonal antibody

MDSC: myeloid-derived suppressor cell – a type of myeloid progenitor immune cell that inhibits immune responses, produces cytokines that promote tumor invasion and metastasis, such as interleukin-6, and suppresses T-cell activation

MHC: major histocompatibility complex – cell surface proteins that bind to antigens and expose them to antigen-presenting cells, thereby facilitating adaptive immune responses

Naive T cell: a mature T cell – developed in the thymus and released into the periphery – that has not yet encountered a specific antigen

NK cells: natural killer cells – a type of T cell that contributes to innate immune responses

NLR: nucleotide-binding oligomerization domain-like receptor – a group of pattern recognition receptors that play key roles in innate immune responses

NOD: nucleotide-binding oligomerization domain

nT_{reg} cells: natural regulatory T cells

Opsonization: labeling of pathogens or other foreign material by enzymes of the complement system, which facilitates phagocytosis by cells of the innate immune system

OX40: Tumor necrosis factor receptor superfamily member 4

PAMP: pathogen-associated molecular pattern – a molecule secreted by a pathogen, such as bacterial lipopolysaccharide, which is recognized by immune cells expressing pattern recognition receptors

PD-1: programmed cell death-1 (receptor) – an immune checkpoint that plays an important role in enabling cancer cells to avoid detection and elimination by the immune system

PD-L1: programmed cell death 1 receptor ligand

Pericytes: a specialized mesenchymal cell type related to smooth muscle cells, that support the tumor endothelium

Phagocytosis: ingestion of pathogens or other foreign material by cells such as macrophages, monocytes and neutrophils

PRR: pattern recognition receptor – proteins present on the surface of inflammatory cells such as macrophages, which recognize foreign proteins (collectively known as pathogen-associated molecular patterns)

Pseudoprogression: an apparent increase in tumor size following the start of immunotherapy, caused by infiltration of reactivated T cells into the tumor, causing inflammation

RECIST: Response Evaluation Criteria in Solid Tumors

T cells: a type of lymphocyte that plays a number of key roles in immune responses

TAA: tumor-associated antigen

TCR: T cell receptor

T_{eff}: effector T cells

TGF-β: transforming growth factor-β – a cytokine that plays an important role in inducing differentiation of regulatory T cells

T_h: helper T cells

TIGIT: T cell immunoreceptor with immunoglobulin and immunoreceptor tyrosine-based inhibitory domains – an immune receptor present on some T cells and natural killer cells

TIL: tumor-infiltrating lymphocyte

TLR: toll-like receptor

TNF: tumor necrosis factor

Toll-like receptor ligands: a group of proteins that play important roles in antigen recognition by the innate immune system

T_{reg}: regulatory T cells

Introduction

Recent advances in immuno-oncology have revolutionized the treatment of cancer. With treatment aimed at modulating the immune system, some patients with incurable advanced cancers may now experience long-term responses and significantly improved survival. This has led to unprecedented accelerated regulatory approvals, with promising therapies already being incorporated into the current standards of care for many tumor types. Although significant challenges remain and many more questions remain unanswered, the field is expected to move at even faster speed.

Today, most oncology professionals need a good understanding of immuno-oncology to practice at the highest level. This includes knowledge of the fundamentals of immunology, cancer immunoediting and the many different types of cancer immunotherapy, including immune checkpoint inhibitors. It is important to grasp the future directions of this evolving field. However, it is difficult to obtain the key facts from the sea of information out there, especially when one has little time.

Whether you are a practicing oncologist, an oncology health professional, a medical student, a cancer researcher or industry professional, *Fast Facts: Immuno-Oncology* provides you with all you need to know about the topic, concisely summarized. The book was especially written so that, after an easy read, you will be well equipped to understand immuno-oncology in the context of your professional work.

1 Components of the immune system

The immune system has evolved to protect the host against infectious agents such as bacteria, viruses and fungi, and to detect and eliminate potentially harmful foreign material. A hallmark of cancer is that tumor cells – which would normally be recognized by the immune system as abnormal – acquire the ability to evade the immune system.[1] Immuno-oncology is a new, multi-faceted and rapidly evolving collection of treatment strategies aimed at harnessing immune processes to target and destroy tumor cells and prolong survival.[2] An understanding of the basic elements of the normal and tumor-altered immune system is therefore key to understanding potential immuno-oncology therapies.

The immune system consists of two components: *innate* immunity and *adaptive* immunity.

- Innate immunity is conferred by mechanisms that are present throughout life, such as the physical barriers to infection provided by the skin and mucous membranes, white blood cells that remove foreign material, and serum proteins such as lysozymes and kinins.
- Adaptive (acquired) immunity is conferred by the formation of antibodies following exposure to foreign material (antigens), and is specific to the particular antigen.

In general, innate immune reactions provide a rapid (within hours) but non-specific initial response to infection or injury, whereas adaptive immune responses are more specific to the foreign antigen and develop over a longer period (Figure 1.1).

Innate immunity

In addition to the physical barrier of skin and membranes, innate immunity is primarily conferred by phagocytic cells derived from stem cells in the bone marrow. The most important of these include macrophages, monocytes and neutrophils, although other cell types, such as natural killer (NK) cells, also play important roles (Table 1.1).

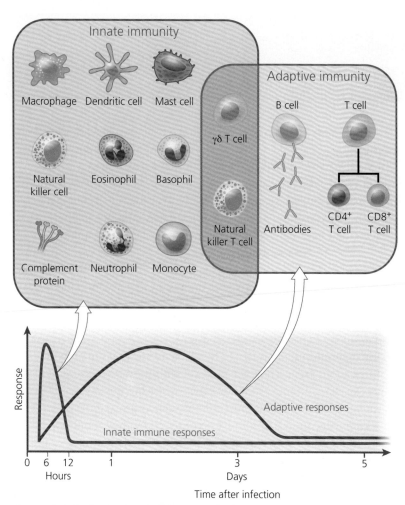

Figure 1.1 The body's initial defenses in the first critical hours of exposure to a new pathogen are non-specific innate immune responses. Pathogens are recognized by a variety of immune cells, as shown here. Adaptive (acquired) immune responses are specific to the particular antigen, and develop over several days.

Phagocytosis. Phagocytes are attracted to foreign material, such as a pathogen, and engulf it in a process known as phagocytosis. The foreign material is then contained inside an endosome, and digested by enzymes and acids contained in organelles known as lysosomes.

TABLE 1.1

Cell types contributing to innate immune responses

• Macrophages	• Dendritic cells
• Monocytes	• Mast cells
• Neutrophils	• Natural killer (NK) cells
• Basophils	• Natural killer (NK) T cells
• Eosinophils	

Phagocytosis is facilitated by the *complement* system (Figure 1.2), a cascade of plasma proteins that:
• form holes in the plasma membranes of pathogens, leading to cell lysis
• label pathogens for destruction by coating the cell surface (opsonization)
• recruit inflammatory cells to sites of infection or injury
• eliminate antigen–antibody complexes.
Following activation, phagocytic cells secrete inflammatory proteins, including cytokines and interleukins, which trigger further recruitment of inflammatory cells to sites of infection and cellular damage.

The role of inflammation in immune responses

Inflammation is a primary immune response to tissue damage resulting from infection or injury. Acute inflammation is triggered by resident cells such as macrophages and dendritic cells, which have receptors on their surfaces known as pattern recognition receptors (PRRs). These recognize and bind to pathogen-associated molecular patterns (PAMPs) on the pathogen cells, resulting in activation of the immune cell and release of inflammatory mediators such as histamine, kinins and prostaglandins, which recruit neutrophils and other phagocytic cells to the damaged tissue. Neutrophils in turn release cytokines that trigger the recruitment of further immune cells. Cytokine release from immune cells leads to the characteristic signs of inflammation:
• redness due to local vasodilatation
• heat (either localized to the site of injury or systemic fever)
• swelling of affected tissues
• pain.

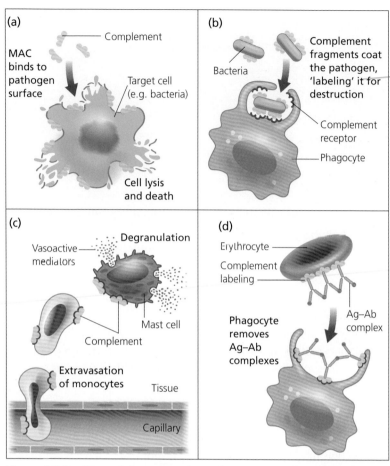

Figure 1.2 Functions of the activated complement system in an innate immune response. (a) The membrane attack complex (MAC) formed by complement activation binds to the surface of a pathogen, disrupting its cell membrane, causing cell lysis and death. (b) The proteolytic complement fragment C3b (also C4b and iC3b) coats the pathogen, in effect 'labeling' it for destruction by the phagocytic cells that express complement receptors that bind to C3b, C4b and iC3b (opsonization). (c) The complement fragments C5a, C4a and C3a induce acute inflammation by, for example, binding to mast cells and inducing degranulation, with the release of vasoactive mediators such as histamine. (d) In the spleen and liver, phagocytic cells remove antigen–antibody (Ag–Ab) complexes from erythrocyte surfaces because of the complement 'labeling' on the immune complex.

Importantly, inflammation is a feature of almost all neoplastic lesions and has been recognized as one of the hallmarks of cancer.[1] To some extent, this reflects an attempt by the immune system to eradicate cancerous tissue, but it is now recognized that inflammation can itself promote tumor growth by various mechanisms. These include:

- production of growth factors, proangiogenic factors and other agents capable of promoting tumor growth
- activation of cell growth patterns leading to high-grade malignancy
- production of reactive oxygen species and other potential mutagens.[1]

Adaptive (acquired) immunity

Adaptive immune responses are primarily mediated by lymphocytes, and may be categorized according to the type of lymphocyte involved:

- cellular (or cell-mediated) immunity is mediated by T cells originating in the thymus
- humoral immunity is mediated by B cells derived from bone marrow.
 In both cases, immune cells are activated following exposure to antigens such as proteins, polysaccharides, lipids or nucleic acids, leading to an immune response directed against specific antigens.

Recognition of self and non-self. A key step in adaptive immunity is the presentation of antigens to immune cells. All cells present surface antigens that are complexed with major histocompatibility complex (MHC) class I proteins, allowing the immune system to distinguish between 'self' and 'non-self'. In addition, however, dendritic cells act as 'professional' antigen-presenting cells (APCs), expressing MHC class I and II proteins that bind to antigens and present them to naive (undifferentiated) T cells (Figure 1.3).

 Major histocompatibility complex is a set of cell surface proteins that bind to antigens derived from pathogens, including tumors, displaying them on the cell surface for recognition by T cells. MHC class I molecules are present on all nucleated cells and platelets, and serve to trigger a cytotoxic T-cell response to the infected cell. MHC class II molecules are only present on specialized APCs such as dendritic cells, and serve to alert the immune system through T helper cells.

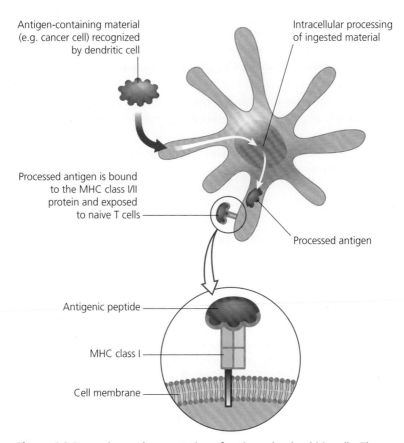

Antigen-containing material
(e.g. cancer cell) recognized
by dendritic cell

Intracellular processing
of ingested material

Processed antigen is bound
to the MHC class I/II
protein and exposed
to naive T cells

Processed antigen

Antigenic peptide

MHC class I

Cell membrane

Figure 1.3 Processing and presentation of antigens by dendritic cells. The major histocompatibility complex (MHC) protein (inset) acts as a recognizable 'scaffold' that presents pieces (peptides) of a foreign protein (antigen) to undifferentiated T cells.

Cellular immunity. Surface T cell receptors (TCRs) are specific to individual antigens, and are activated when the TCR binds to the appropriate antigen. The availability of T cells to respond to the wide variety of potential antigens is achieved through extensive random rearrangements in the *TCR* gene during T-cell development in the thymus. Inevitably, such random rearrangements will occasionally produce TCRs that bind to 'self' antigens; in this situation, the T cells are eliminated or deactivated in a process known as self-tolerance. If this process is incomplete, autoimmune diseases may arise.

T cells recognize their target antigens as protein sequences presented on the surface of APCs in association with MHC molecules.

CD4+ T cells, which are subdivided into helper (T_h) and regulatory (T_{reg}) T cells, recognize antigens bound to MHC class II molecules. Activation of T_h cells, which requires a weaker stimulus than for cytotoxic T cells, leads to cytokine release that affects multiple immune cells including APCs. There are two types of CD4+ T cell responses.

- Th1 responses are primarily directed against intracellular pathogens, and are characterized by production of interferon (IFN)-γ, induction of opsonization, and antibody production by B cells.
- Th2 responses are effective against extracellular bacteria and parasites, and are characterized by production of interleukin (IL)-4 and -5.

T_{reg} cells mainly regulate and suppress the immune response of naive and effector T cells through a variety of cytokine and signaling mechanisms, including transforming growth factor (TGF)-β and IL-10. T_{reg} cells regulate the immune response to common environmental allergens and prevent the development of atopy or undesirable inflammation. However, their role in maintenance of peripheral tolerance is also used by cancers to evade the immune system.

CD8+ cytotoxic T cells (also known as killer T cells) are activated by antigens from intracellular pathogens presented on MHC class I molecules. Activation of these cells triggers a process known as *clonal selection*, during which the T cells proliferate to produce a population of effector T cells (T_{eff}). These cells recognize cells with a unique MHC class I–antigen complex, and release enzymes and toxins that lyse the cell membrane and induce programmed cell death (apoptosis). To prevent extensive tissue damage during an infection, activation of CD8+ cells requires three signals (Figure 1.4):

- binding of the antigen to the TCR
- binding of the MHC class I or II molecules to accessory CD8 or CD4 molecules, respectively, on the T cell
- co-regulatory (co-stimulatory and co-inhibitory) signals resulting from binding of CD80 (B7-1) and CD28 on the APC and T cell: binding of CD80 (B7-1) on the APC to T cell CD28 leads to a positive signal, causing the T cell to kill cells bearing the relevant antigen, whereas binding of CD80 (B7-1) on the APC to CTLA-4 (cytotoxic T-lymphocyte-associated protein 4) on the T cell results in a negative signal, preventing the T cell from killing antigen-bearing cells.

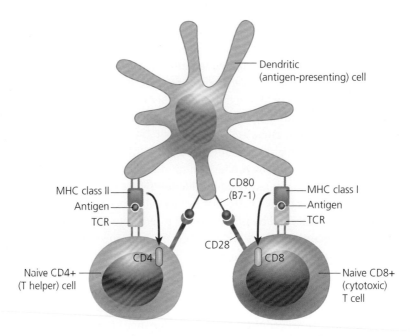

Figure 1.4 Activation of cytotoxic T cells. CD8+ cytotoxic T cells are activated by antigens from intracellular pathogens presented on major histocompatibility complex (MHC) class I molecules. CD4+ cells recognize antigens presented on MHC class II molecules. Activation requires three signals: the binding of the antigen to the T-cell receptor (TCR); binding of the MHC class I or II molecules to accessory CD8 or CD4 molecules, respectively, on the T cell; and co-regulatory signals from the binding of CD80 (B7-1) and CD28 on the antigen-presenting (dendritic) cell and T cell. Adapted from Messerschmidt et al. 2016.

Humoral immunity involves the production in B cells of antibodies (immunoglobulins) against specific antigens. In contrast to T cells, where the antigen is processed intracellularly before being expressed on the cell surface in association with MHC molecules, B cells recognize the native, unprocessed, form of the antigen.

The B cell receptor (BCR) consists of an antibody that recognizes a specific antigen. Upon activation by binding of the antigen to the BCR, B cells differentiate into short-lived antibody-producing cells (plasma cells) (Figure 1.5). The antibodies bind to the antigen, rendering it more susceptible to phagocytosis and triggering the complement system.

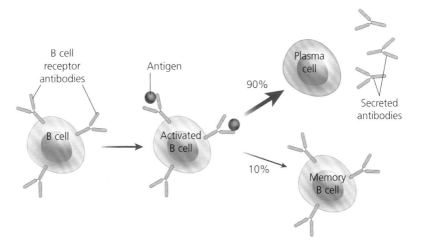

Figure 1.5 Activation and differentiation of B cells. Binding of the antigen to the B cell receptor activates the B cell. Most B cells then differentiate into short-lived antibody-producing cells (plasma cells). Approximately 10% differentiate into long-lived antigen-specific memory B cells.

Once the antigen has been cleared, the plasma cells are eliminated via programmed cell death (apoptosis). However, approximately 10% of activated B cells differentiate into long-lived antigen-specific memory B cells (see Figure 1.5); this allows a rapid immune response to be mounted in the event of re-exposure to the antigen.

Full activation and differentiation of B cells requires an additional co-stimulatory signal, from either T_h cells or T cell-independent mechanisms such as toll-like receptor ligands (a group of proteins that play important roles in antigen recognition by the innate immune system).

Inter-relationship between innate and adaptive immunity

There is a close inter-relationship between the innate and adaptive immune systems, which is mediated via cytokines and other messengers (Figure 1.6). One well-characterized function of NK cells is antibody-dependent cell-mediated cytotoxicity (ADCC). NK cells, which are part of the innate immune system, cooperate with the adaptive humoral immunity through binding of the Fc portion of antigen-specific immunoglobulin (Ig) G. NK cells are activated

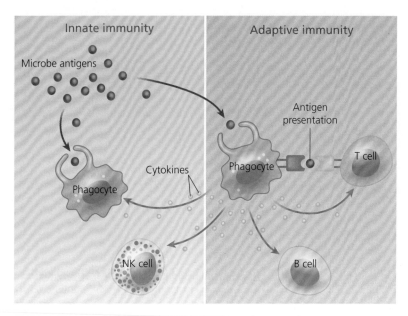

Figure 1.6 Inter-relationship between innate and acquired immune systems, mediated by cytokines and other messengers. NK, natural killer cells. Adapted from https://clinicalgate.com/cells-tissues-and-organs-of-the-immune-system.

through the cross-linking of CD16 on the NK cell surface and the Fc portion of IgG, and consequently eliminate the target through the release of lytic granular contents. Other effector cells from the innate immune system, such as macrophages, neutrophils and eosinophils, can also mediate ADCC through similar mechanisms.

Development of immune tolerance

Immune tolerance is a state in which the immune system is unresponsive to a stimulus that would normally provoke an immune response. It is an important mechanism by which tumor cells evade the immune system.

Immune tolerance may be central or peripheral, depending on where it is induced:
- central tolerance is induced in the thymus and bone marrow
- peripheral tolerance is induced in lymph nodes or other tissues.

Central tolerance is the principal mechanism by which the immune system learns to distinguish between 'self' and 'non-self'. Maturing T and B lymphocytes in the thymus and bone marrow, respectively, are presented with self-antigens; cells bearing receptors for these antigens are removed by apoptosis or by induction of an inactive state known as anergy. Some autoreactive B cells may be retained in a state in which they do not respond to stimulation of their receptors. Conversely, some weakly autoreactive T cells may differentiate into natural regulatory T cells (nT_{reg}), which act in the periphery to diminish potential T cell autoreactivity (see below).

Peripheral tolerance plays a key role in preventing hyperreactivity of the immune system in response to environmental agents such as allergens or gut microbes. A number of mechanisms contribute to peripheral tolerance, primarily involving regulation of T-cell populations, particularly CD4+ T_h cells.

- Autoreactive T cells that are not eliminated in the thymus can be neutralized by nT_{reg} cells, as described above.
- Following repeated exposure to antigens, naive CD4+ T_h cells differentiate into induced T_{reg} cells, a process mediated by IL-12 production following T-cell activation, and by TGF-β secreted by APCs.
- Peripheral tolerance may also be mediated by other T-cell populations resembling T_{reg} cells, such as TR1 cells that express IL-10, and TH3 cells that secrete TGF-β.
- Some dendritic cells are able to produce indoleamine 2,3-disoxygenase (IDO), which depletes intracellular supplies of tryptophan, an amino acid needed for T-cell proliferation.

In addition to these T-cell mechanisms, peripheral tolerance may result from expression in B cells of CD22, a non-specific receptor inhibitor that decreases activation of BCRs, and by production of IL-10 and TGF-β in B cells.

Key points – components of the immune system

- The immune system has two components: *innate* immunity, involving mechanisms present throughout life, and *adaptive (acquired)* immunity, which is conferred by immune responses following exposure to an antigen, and is specific to that antigen.
- Innate immunity is primarily conferred by phagocytic cells derived from stem cells in the bone marrow, principally macrophages, monocytes and neutrophils.
- There are two forms of adaptive immunity: cellular immunity mediated by T cells originating in the thymus, and humoral immunity mediated by B cells originating in the bone marrow.
- In cellular immunity, T cells recognize their target antigens as protein sequences presented on the surface of antigen-presenting cells (APCs) in association with major histocompatibility complex (MHC) molecules.
  - Activation of CD4+ T cells leads to cytokine release that affects multiple immune cells, including APCs.
  - Activation of CD8+ cytotoxic T cells triggers clonal selection, during which the T cells proliferate to produce a population of effector T cells, which release enzymes and toxins that lyse the membrane of antigen-bearing cells and induce programmed cell death (apoptosis).
- Humoral immunity involves the production by B cells of antibodies against specific antigens.
- Immune tolerance is a state in which the immune system is unresponsive to a stimulus that would normally provoke an immune response. This may be central or peripheral, depending on where tolerance develops. Immune tolerance is an important mechanism by which tumor cells evade the immune system.

References

1 Hanahan D, Weinberg RA. Hallmarks of cancer: the next generation. *Cell* 2011;144:646–74.

2 Kamta J, Chaar M, Ande A et al. Advancing cancer therapy with present and emerging immuno-oncology approaches. *Front Oncol* 2017;7:64.

Further reading

Messerschmidt JL, Prendergast GC, Messerschmidt GL. How cancers escape immune destruction and mechanisms of action for the new significantly active immune therapies: helping nonimmunologists decipher recent advances. *Oncologist* 2016;21:233–43.

2 How cancers evade the immune system

The possibility of harnessing the immune system to attack cancer cells was first proposed over 100 years ago,[1] but effective immunotherapies have until recently proved elusive because of the ability of cancer cells to evade the immune system. Indeed, as noted in the previous chapter, this ability can be considered one of the defining features of cancer.[2]

The cancer immunity cycle

The response of the immune system to cancer cells is a cyclical process (Figure 2.1) that may in principle be self-perpetuating, leading to a heightened immune response. Initially, cancer cells are detected by natural killer (NK) cells, which interact with specific ligands on the cancer cell surface, leading to the destruction of the cancer cells. This causes the release of cancer antigens that bind to dendritic cells or other antigen-presenting cells (APCs), leading to cytokine secretion by APCs and priming the activation of T cells in lymphoid tissue. These cytotoxic T cells are transported to the tumor, where they bind to major histocompatibility complex (MHC) class I proteins on the cancer cell surface and kill the target cancer cells. This in turn leads to further release of antigens, thereby amplifying the immune response. However, each step in the process has multiple regulators – both positive and negative. The negative regulators can set up feedback loops that diminish or block the immune response. In addition to allowing the tumor cell to evade immune attack, these mechanisms may actually facilitate tumor progression.

Immunoediting of cancer cells: the 'three Es'

The recognition that the immune system may both suppress and promote tumor growth has led to a shift in attention away from immunosurveillance (with a focus on recognition and elimination of cancer cells) to *immunoediting* (which encompasses both immunosurveillance and pro-proliferative mechanisms). Depending on the type of cancer and the characteristics of the individual patient,

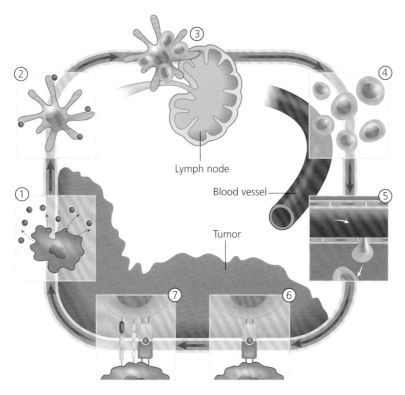

Figure 2.1 The cancer immunity cycle.
(1) Destruction of cancer cells leads to the release of cancer antigens.
(2) The cancer antigens bind to dentritic cells or other APCs.
(3) The APCs then secrete cytokines, which activate T cells in lymphoid tissue.
(4) The activated (cytotoxic) T cells are transported in the blood to the tumor.
(5) The cytotoxic T cells infiltrate the tumor bed.
(6) At the tumor, cytotoxic T cells bind to MHC class I proteins on the surface of cancer cells.
(7) The cancer cells are destroyed, leading to the release of cancer antigens (step 1 again).
APC, antigen-presenting cell; MHC, major histocompatibility complex.
Adapted from Chen et al. 2013.

tumor immunoediting can be governed by at least three aspects, known collectively as the 'three Es': Elimination, Equilibrium and Escape (Table 2.1).[3,4]

TABLE 2.1

The three Es of tumor immunoediting

Elimination	Some cancer cells are recognized as altered by the immune system, and are destroyed.
Equilibrium	Some cancer cells persist, but the immune response is sufficient to prevent proliferation. Eventually, however, selective pressure leads to a predominance of cells that are able to avoid the immune response, leading to...
Evasion	Resistant cancer cells acquire the ability to evade detection or elimination by immune cells, leading to clinically apparent disease.

How tumors evade immune attack

Tumor cells can block immune responses in a number of ways.

- Cancer cell antigens may not be recognized by dendritic cells or APCs.
- Cancer antigens may be treated as self-antigens, rather than foreign, leading to regulatory T cell (T_{reg}) responses rather than cancer-specific effector responses.
- T cells may not be trafficked to the tumor, or are prevented from infiltrating the tumor.
- Factors in the tumor microenvironment (see page 30) may suppress effector T (T_{eff}) cells.

Two principal mechanisms by which these effects are achieved involve the programmed cell death-1 (PD-1) and the cytotoxic T lymphocyte-associated antigen 4 (CTLA-4) immune checkpoints. Both of these are important therapeutic targets in immuno-oncology (see Chapter 4).

The PD-1 receptor pathway. The PD-1 receptor on the surface of T cells plays an important role in regulating the recruitment and activation of T cells, and overexpression of this receptor's ligand, PD-L1, by cancer cells has been reported in several types of cancer, including melanoma and cancers of the lung, kidney, head and neck, and colon.[5] Binding of this receptor to its ligand, PD-L1, can affect the immune response to cancer cells in two ways.

- In the lymph nodes, overexpression of PD-L1 in tumor-infiltrating immune cells can prevent the priming and activation of new cytotoxic T cells, and subsequently prevent recruitment of these immune cells to the tumor.
- Within the tumor microenvironment, up-regulation of PD-L1 on cancer cells and immune cells such as macrophages, dendritic cells and T cells leads to deactivation of cytotoxic T cells.

In both cases, binding of PD-L1 to PD-1 on the surface of T cells results in the development of T-cell tolerance, with reduced T-cell proliferation, decreased cytokine expression and impaired antigen recognition (Figure 2.2).

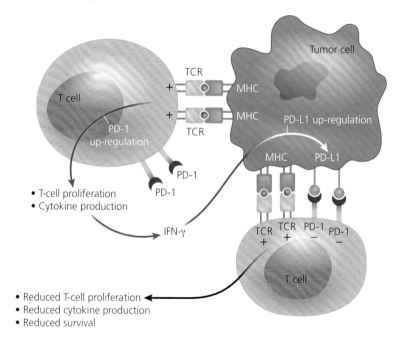

Figure 2.2 Effects of the PD-1 receptor on T-cell function. Binding of PD-1 on the surface of T cells to its ligand (PD-L1) on tumor cells leads to the development of T-cell tolerance, with reduced T-cell proliferation, decreased cytokine expression and impaired antigen recognition. IFN-γ, interferon-γ; MHC, major histocompatibility complex; PD-1, programmed cell death (receptor); PD-L1, PD-1 receptor ligand; TCR, T-cell receptor. Adapted from Buchbinder et al. 2016.[6]

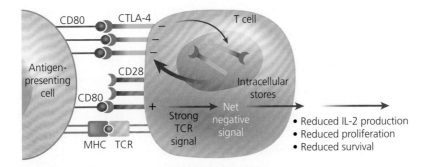

Figure 2.3 Effects of CTLA-4 on T-cell function. Binding of CD80 (B7-1) on the antigen-presenting cell to CTLA-4 on the T cell leads to decreased production of interleukin (IL)-2 by T cells and impaired T-cell proliferation and survival. CD, cluster of differentiation; CTLA-4, cytotoxic T lymphocyte-associated antigen; MHC, major histocompatibility complex; TCR, T-cell receptor. Adapted from Buchbinder et al. 2016.[6]

The CTLA-4 pathway. As described in Chapter 1, activation of cytotoxic CD8+ T cells requires positive co-regulatory (or co-stimulatory) signals resulting from binding of CD80 (B7-1) and CD28 on APCs and T cells. On the other hand, binding of CD80 (B7-1) on the APC to CTLA-4 on the T cell results in a negative signal, leading to decreased interleukin (IL)-2 production by T cells and impaired T-cell proliferation and survival (Figure 2.3). Consequently, CTLA-4 is an important immune checkpoint and target for cancer immunotherapy.

Differences between the PD-1/PD-L1 and CTLA-4 pathways have implications for their use as therapeutic targets in immuno-oncology.[7] In particular, the effects of PD-1 are largely confined to the tumor site: expression of PD-L1 is low in non-cancerous tissue. Furthermore, therapies acting on PD-1/PD-L1 have the potential to reset tumor-related alterations in the immune system while leaving normal peripheral tolerance to self-antigens unaffected. These differences between the two pathways suggest that combined PD-1/PD-L1 and CTLA-4 blockade might have synergistic anti-tumor effects: CTLA-4 blockade allows activation and proliferation of more T-cell populations while reducing T_{reg}-mediated immunosuppression, and PD-1/PD-L1

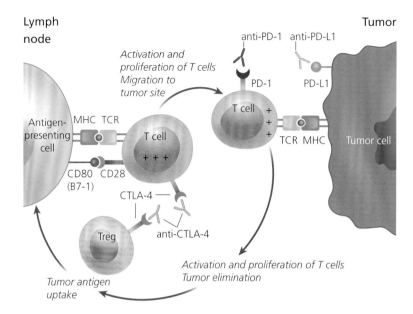

Figure 2.4 Potential synergistic anti-tumor effect of combined PD-1 and CTLA-4 blockade. CTLA-4, cytotoxic T lymphocyte-associated antigen-4; MHC, major histocompatibility complex; PD-1, programmed cell death-1 (receptor). PD-L1, PD-1 receptor ligand; TCR, T-cell receptor; T_{reg}: regulatory T cell. Adapted from Buchbinder et al. 2016.[6]

blockade restores the activity of quiescent T cells (Figure 2.4). It has also been suggested that therapies directed against PD-1/PD-L1 should be termed ***tumor site immune modulation therapy***, to distinguish this approach from CTLA-4 blockade.[7]

Other inhibitory receptors on T cells, including TIM-3, BTLA, VISTA and LAG-3, could represent additional targets for immunotherapeutics (Figure 2.5). In addition, the stimulation of agonistic receptors on T cells promotes activation of T cells. Some of these include CD28, OX40, GITR, CD-137, CD27 and HVEM. Other molecules such as TIGIT (T-cell immunoreceptor with immunoglobulin and immunoreceptor tyrosine-based inhibitory [ITIM] domains), which have co-inhibitory roles with PD-1 and also affect T-cell activity, can also be targeted. Further understanding of the biology of immune regulation in cancer will define optimal targets and combinations for therapeutic interventions.

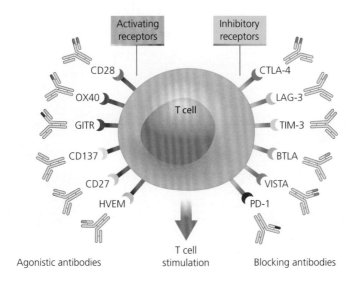

Figure 2.5 Activating and inhibitory receptors on T cells.

The importance of the tumor microenvironment

Tumors are complex structures consisting of multiple cell types that create a constantly evolving immunosuppressive microenvironment (Figure 2.6). This microenvironment can inhibit immune responses and promote tumor growth through a number of mechanisms (Table 2.2).

In addition to the cancer cells themselves, a number of different cell types may contribute to the tumor microenvironment (see Figure 2.6). These include:

- cancer stem cells (CSCs), which are resistant to commonly used chemotherapy agents, and may contribute to disease recurrence after apparently successful tumor debulking
- endothelial cells, particularly those in the tumor blood vessels, which play an important role in tumor angiogenesis
- pericytes, a specialized mesenchymal cell type related to smooth muscle cells, that support the tumor endothelium
- immune inflammatory cells, including cells with tumor-promoting activities, such as macrophage subtypes, mast cells and neutrophils, and partially differentiated myeloid progenitor cells
- cancer-associated fibroblasts
- stem and progenitor cells in the tumor stroma.

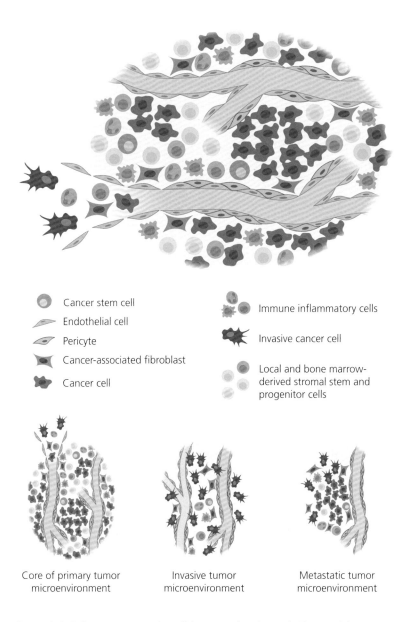

Cancer stem cell

Endothelial cell

Pericyte

Cancer-associated fibroblast

Cancer cell

Immune inflammatory cells

Invasive cancer cell

Local and bone marrow-derived stromal stem and progenitor cells

Core of primary tumor microenvironment

Invasive tumor microenvironment

Metastatic tumor microenvironment

Figure 2.6 Cell types present in solid tumors (top image). The resulting immunosuppressive microenvironment (bottom images) is constantly evolving. Adapted from Hanahan and Weinberg 2011.[2]

TABLE 2.2

Mechanisms contributing to an immunosuppressive tumor microenvironment[8]

Immune exclusion	• Altered chemokine expression to impair T-cell trafficking to tumor site
	• Physical or metabolic barriers
Modulation of suppressive immune cells	• Induction of T_{reg}-mediated immune tolerance:
	– induction of T_{reg} differentiation by secretion of TGF-β
	– recruitment of circulating T_{reg} by secretion of CCL22
	• Decreased transformation of myeloid-derived suppressor cells into dendritic cells
Immunosuppression through direct interactions with T cells	• Over-expression of negative co-regulatory molecules such as PD-1 and CEACAM1

CCL22, C–C motif chemokine 22; CEACAM1, carcinoembryonic antigen-related cell adhesion molecule 1; PD-1, programmed cell death-1 receptor; TGF-β, transforming growth factor-β; T_{reg}, regulatory T cells.

Goals of immuno-oncology therapies

The aim of immuno-oncology therapies is to restore the ability of the immune system to recognize and eliminate cancer cells. This can potentially be achieved by either:
- activating the immune system directly, for example, with vaccines
- inhibiting the suppression of the immune system by tumors.

Key points – how cancers evade the immune system

- The immune response to the presence of cancer cells is a cyclical process that is potentially self-propagating. However, the existence of numerous negative regulators allows tumor cells to evade the immune system.
- Tumor immunoediting has three components, known as the 'three Es': elimination, equilibrium and evasion:
  - during the initial elimination phase, some cancer cells are recognized as altered by the immune system and are destroyed
  - during the equilibrium phase, some cancer cells persist, but the immune response is sufficient to prevent proliferation
  - eventually, however, selective pressure leads to a predominance of cells that are able to avoid the immune response – escape.
- The immune checkpoint molecules PD-1 and CTLA-4 are key factors in the ability of tumor cells to evade the immune system. However, there are multiple other potential targets, some of which have inhibitory activity and others agonistic activity in T-cell activation.
- Solid tumors consist of multiple cell types that together contribute to the development of a microenvironment that favors tumor growth and evasion of the immune system.

Key references

1 Kreamer KM. Immune checkpoint blockade: a new paradigm in treating advanced cancer. *J Adv Pract Oncol* 2014;5:418–31.

2 Hanahan D, Weinberg RA. Hallmarks of cancer: the next generation. *Cell* 2011;144:646–74.

3 Schreiber RD, Old LJ, Smyth MJ. Cancer immunoediting: integrating immunity's roles in cancer suppression and promotion. *Science* 2011;331:1565–70.

4 Dunn GP, Old LJ, Schreiber RD. The three Es of cancer immunoediting. *Annu Rev Immunol* 2004;22:329–60.

5. Herbst RS, Soria J-C, Kowanetz M et al. Predictive correlates of response to the anti-PD-L1 antibody MPDL3280A in cancer patients. *Nature* 2014;515:563–7.

6 Buchbinder EI, Desai A. CTLA-4 and PD-1 pathways: similarities, differences, and implications of their inhibition. *Am J Clin Oncol* 2016;39:98–106.

7 Wang J, Yuan R, Song W et al. PD-1, PD-L1 (B7-H1) and tumor-site immune modulation therapy: the historical perspective. *J Hematol Oncol* 2017;10:34.

8 Hanahan D, Weinberg RA. Hallmarks of cancer: the next generation. *Cell* 2011;144:646–74.

Further reading

Chen DS, Mellman I. Oncology meets immunology: the cancer-immunity cycle. *Immunity* 2013; 39:1–10.

Finn OJ. Immuno-oncology: understanding the function and dysfunction of the immune system in cancer. *Ann Oncol* 2012;23(Suppl 8):viii6–9.

Robainas M, Otano R, Bueno S, Ait-Oudhia S. Understanding the role of PD-L1/PD1 pathway blockade and autophagy in cancer therapy. *Onco Targets Ther* 2017;10:1803–7.

3 How cancer immunotherapy works

In the context of cancer, the term immunotherapy encompasses a variety of approaches, targeting diverse immunologic targets.

The history of immuno-oncology

The concept of immuno-oncology dates back more than 100 years, to 1893 (Figure 3.1). In that year, William Coley, an American surgeon and cancer researcher, observed remission of cancer in patients with postoperative bacterial infections, and suggested that activation of the immune system must play a role in combating cancer.[1,2] Subsequently,

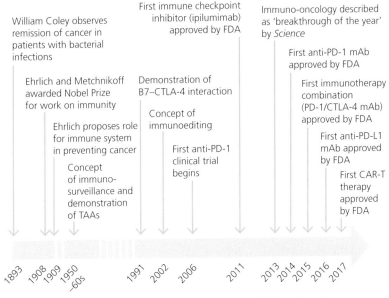

Figure 3.1 The history of immuno-oncology. CAR-T, chimeric antigen receptor-expressing T cell; CTLA-4, cytotoxic T-lymphocyte-associated protein 4; FDA, Food and Drug Administration; mAb, monoclonal antibody; PD-1, programmed cell death-1 receptor; PD-L1, ligand for PD-1; TAA, tumor-associated antigen.[1–9]

in 1909, Paul Ehrlich suggested that the immune system must play an important role in preventing the development of cancer.[3] However, it was not until the mid-20th century when Lewis Thomas and Frank MacFarlane Burnet hypothesized that the immune system is capable of eliminating cancerous cells through a process known as immune surveillance, and that this process depends on recognition of tumor-associated antigens by the immune system.[4,5] Subsequently, through the laboratory work of Lloyd Old and Robert Schreiber, the concept of immune surveillance has evolved into 'immunoediting', reflecting the ability of tumor cells to evade the immune system.[6] Increasing understanding of the underlying mechanisms of immunoediting has identified numerous potential therapeutic targets, some of which – notably immune checkpoint inhibition as first demonstrated by James Allison in the 1990s – are already yielding promising results in clinical practice.[7,8] Indeed, in 2013, cancer immunotherapy was cited as the 'breakthrough of the year' by the journal *Science*.[9]

What types of tumor are potentially susceptible to immuno-oncology?

Clearly, the potential sensitivity of a given cancer to immuno-oncology therapies will depend on the ability of the tumor to trigger an immune response (immunogenicity). Cancer is characterized by an accumulation of genetic mutations, many of which result in the expression of cancer-specific antigens that can bind to major histocompatibility complex (MHC) class I molecules on the cancer cell surface.[10] These antigen–MHC complexes can be recognized by cytotoxic CD8+ lymphocytes, that, if activated, could potentially mount an immune response against the tumor. As a result, tumors with high somatic mutation rates may be more susceptible to immuno-oncology therapies than those with lower mutation rates.

Somatic mutation rates differ markedly, both between tumor types and within an individual tumor type: the rate may vary more than 1000-fold between tumors with the highest and lowest rates (Figure 3.2). The highest rates are seen in cancers of the skin, lung, bladder and stomach, while the lowest are seen in hematologic and pediatric cancers. It is noteworthy that the highest rates occur in tumors that are induced by carcinogens such as tobacco smoke or ultraviolet light.

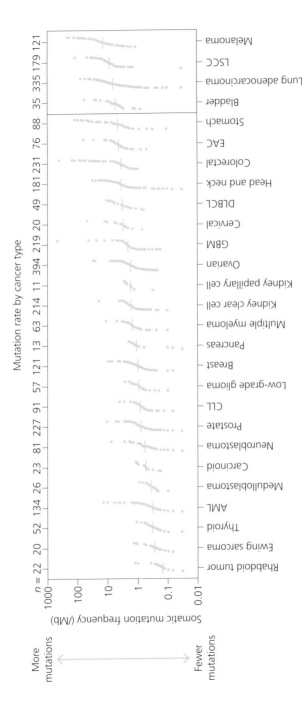

Figure 3.2 Somatic mutation rates in different tumors. Each dot corresponds to a tumor–normal pair: the vertical position indicates the total frequency of somatic mutations. Tumors with the highest mutation rates (right-hand side of the figure) would be expected to be most susceptible to immuno-oncology therapies. AML, acute myeloid leukemia; CLL, chronic lymphocytic leukemia; DLBCL, diffuse large B-cell lymphoma; EAC, esophageal adenocarcinoma; GBM, glioblastoma multiforme; LSCC, lung squamous cell carcinoma. Reproduced with permission from Lawrence et al. 2013.[11]

37

Potential targets for cancer immunotherapy

A variety of cancer immunotherapy strategies are currently being investigated, or have already entered clinical practice. These are conventionally classified as passive or active immunotherapies, according to their ability to activate an immune response against tumor cells (Table 3.1), although this classification does not adequately reflect the complexity of drug–host–tumor interactions.[12] As a result, it has been suggested that immunotherapies should be classified according to their antigen specificity; however, even therapies initially directed against a single antigen may eventually become responsive to multiple antigens, a phenomenon known as epitope spreading.[12]

Passive immunotherapies

Tumor-targeting monoclonal antibodies. Monoclonal antibodies (mAbs) that specifically target malignant cells are among the best characterized forms of cancer immunotherapy.[12]

TABLE 3.1

Potential types of cancer immunotherapy

Active immunotherapies	Passive immunotherapies
• Anticancer vaccines (preventative and therapeutic)	• Tumor-targeting monoclonal antibodies
• Immunostimulatory cytokines	• Adoptive cell transfer
• Antibodies to proinflammatory cytokines	• Oncolytic viruses
• Immunomodulatory monoclonal antibodies	
• Inhibitors of immunosuppressant metabolism	
• Pattern recognition receptor agonists	
• Immunogenic cell death inducers	

These may act in a number of ways, including:
- inhibition of signaling pathways in tumor cells
- delivery of conjugated cytotoxins or radionuclides to tumor sites
- opsonization of tumor cells and activation of antibody-dependent cell-mediated cytotoxicity (ADCC), antibody-dependent phagocytosis and complement-mediated cytotoxicity
- bispecific T-cell engagers (BiTEs®; Amgen) consisting of single-chain variable fragments from two antibodies targeting a tumor-associated antigen (TAA) and a T-cell surface antigen.

Examples of mAbs that act via these processes are shown in Table 3.2.

Adoptive cell transfer (ACT) is a form of cell-based cancer immunotherapy in which circulating or tumor-infiltrating lymphocytes are collected from the patient, modified ex vivo as necessary to attack specific neoantigens, and reinfused into the patient following lymphodepletion and conditioning (Figure 3.3).

TABLE 3.2

Mechanisms of anti-tumor activity of monoclonal antibodies

Mechanism	Example	Therapeutic target	Indication(s)
Specific inhibition of tumor cell signaling	Cetuximab	EGFR	Head and neck cancer Colorectal cancer
Conjugation with toxin or radionuclide	Trastuzumab emtansine (T-DM1)	HER2	Breast cancer
Opsonization of cancer cells	Rituximab	CD20	Chronic lymphocytic leukemia
BiTE	Blinatumomab	CD19/CD3	B cell acute lymphoblastic leukemia

BiTE®, bispecific T-cell engager; EGFR, epidermal growth factor receptor; HER2, human epidermal growth factor receptor 2; TNF, tumor necrosis factor.

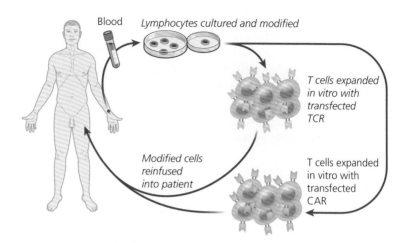

Blood · Lymphocytes cultured and modified

T cells expanded in vitro with transfected TCR

T cells expanded in vitro with transfected CAR

Modified cells reinfused into patient

Figure 3.3 Principles of adoptive cell transfer (ACT). Circulating or tumor-infiltrating lymphocytes are collected from the patient, modified ex vivo as necessary to attack specific neoantigens, and reinfused into the patient following lymphodepletion and conditioning. CAR, chimeric antigen receptor; GM-CSF, granulocyte macrophage colony-stimulating factor; TCR, T-cell receptor. Adapted from Kamta et al. 2017.[1]

Response rates of 80–90% have been achieved with ACT in hematologic cancers, but at present this approach is only available in a few specialized centers.[13]

CAR-T therapy. A form of ACT that is currently attracting considerable attention is the use of chimeric antigen receptor-expressing T (CAR-T) cells. Such T cells are genetically modified to express a transmembrane protein consisting of a synthetic T-cell receptor that targets a predetermined antigen expressed by the tumor. Following infusion of these cells, the patient's immune system actively surveys and engages specific cancer cells that express the antigen. Promising clinical trial results have been achieved with this approach in patients with CD19-positive B-cell hematologic malignancies.[14,15]

Later generations of CAR-T cells included additional co-stimulatory domains to optimize cell activation, and further modifications produced 'armored CAR-T cells', which have been optimized to secrete cytokines or express ligands that offer enhanced efficacy in a hostile tumor microenvironment. Clinical trials are ongoing in patients with various hematologic malignancies and solid tumors, and an important landmark has now been reached with the first approval of a CAR-T therapy. The US Food and Drug Administration (FDA) has approved Kymriah™ (tisagenlecleucel, formerly CTL019) intravenous infusion for the treatment of patients up to 25 years of age with B-cell precursor acute lymphoblastic leukemia (ALL) that is refractory or in second or later relapse, based on an 82% remission rate in a multicenter Phase II registration trial.[16]

Oncolytic viruses are non-pathogenic viruses that specifically infect cancer cells. Such viruses may kill cancer cells in two ways:
- an innate cytopathic effect resulting from overloaded cell metabolism in response to viral infection
- expression of potentially lethal gene products.

To date, Imlygic™ (T-VEC/talimogene laherparepvec) – a genetically engineered oncolytic herpes simplex viral strain that can be injected directly into locally advanced unresectable melanoma tumors – is the only oncolytic virus therapy approved by the US FDA and European Medicines Agency, based on the results of a positive Phase III randomized controlled trial.[17] Clinical trials of T-VEC are ongoing for a variety of cancers, either alone or in combination with immune checkpoint inhibitors.

Active immunotherapies

Preventative antiviral vaccines. Viruses are involved in the development of a range of malignancies (Table 3.3), and such associations are likely to increase as new links between viral infection and cancer are established. These relationships also create the potential for antiviral vaccines to be used to prevent cancer. The best developed of these are the hepatitis B vaccine and vaccines against subtypes of human papillomavirus (HPV) that cause approximately 70% of cervical cancer cases. Data from Taiwan, where there has been mandated universal vaccination of infants against hepatitis B since 1984, have demonstrated reductions in the incidence of both hepatitis B and hepatocellular cancer.[18] Data for the preventive effects of HPV vaccination are preliminary, although modeling has suggested that this will be a highly successful and cost-effective means of

TABLE 3.3

Viruses implicated in cancer development

Virus	Cancer type
Hepatitis B/C	Hepatocellular carcinoma
Epstein–Barr virus	Nasopharyngeal cancer, Burkitt's lymphoma
Human papillomavirus	Cervical cancer, anal cancer, squamous cell carcinoma of neck and head
Human herpes virus 8	Kaposi's sarcoma
Human T-lymphotrophic virus-1	Adult T cell leukemia/lymphoma
Merkel cell polyomavirus	Merkel cell carcinoma
Human immunodeficiency virus	Multiple malignancies

preventing HPV-associated malignancies, especially in low-income populations with high incidence of cervical and head and neck cancers.[19]

Therapeutic vaccines

Dendritic cell-based immunotherapies. Typically, dendritic cell-based immunotherapies involve the isolation of monocytes from the patient or donor, and amplification and differentiation ex vivo in the presence of agents such as granulocyte macrophage colony-stimulating factor (GM-CSF) to induce dendritic cell maturation. The activated dendritic cells are then exposed to a source of TAAs, or mRNA coding for TAAs, and reinfused into the patient. Alternatively, dendritic cells may be allowed to fuse with inactivated cancer cells ex vivo, to create a hybrid known as a dendritome. In both cases, the dendritic cells become loaded with TAAs or TAA mRNA, thereby priming the immune system to mount a response against the relevant antigens.

There is currently no consensus on the optimal approach to dendritic cell-based immunotherapy.[20] To date, only one cell-based product containing dendritic cells has been approved: Sipuleucel-T™

was approved by the FDA in 2010 for the treatment of asymptomatic or minimally symptomatic metastatic castration-resistant prostate cancer, based on a positive Phase III randomized controlled trial.[21] The cost–benefit ratio for this vaccine has been questioned and limits its widespread use.

Peptide- and DNA-based vaccines. Anticancer vaccines could potentially be either peptide-based or DNA-based.

- With peptide-based vaccines, the patient is exposed to TAA peptides, together with adjuvants such as Bacillus Calmette–Guérin (BCG – see below) or lipopolysaccharide (LPS) to stimulate an immune response.
- With DNA-based vaccines, TAAs are encoded into a bacterial plasmid which is injected into the patient and taken up by native cells, including antigen-presenting cells (APCs); the APCs can then produce the antigen themselves to trigger an immune response.

At the time of publication, one of the most widely investigated peptide-based vaccines is the gp (glycoprotein) 100 vaccine for the treatment of metastatic melanoma. This product has been investigated in several clinical trials but the results have been conflicting: in trials that have shown clinical benefit, the vaccine was typically administered with another immuno-oncology therapy such as interleukin (IL)-2 or an immune checkpoint inhibitor.[1] Similarly, no DNA-based vaccine has yet been shown to be beneficial in clinical trials.

Whole-cell tumor vaccines are another potential anticancer vaccination. In this approach, cells are removed from the tumor and inactivated by exposure to ultraviolet radiation, freeze-thawing or heat shock, leading to the release of antigens that will subsequently be recognized by APCs. The attenuated tumor cells are then combined with an appropriate adjuvant and injected back into the patient, triggering an immune response. Whole-cell vaccines have the advantage that the patient is exposed to the full range of TAAs expressed in the tumor, whereas protein-based or DNA-based vaccines involve only a limited number of antigens.

Uncertainties with therapeutic vaccines include their safety and efficacy, although clinical trial safety data look reassuring. Many other questions on optimizing efficacy remain.[22,23]

- Where do they fit in the current treatment paradigm since the advent of effective therapeutic antibodies?

- What is their optimal clinical use: the treatment of advanced disease or (more likely) as a postoperative adjuvant therapy?
- What is the most effective immune-stimulatory adjuvant? Some of the more effective adjuvants, including BCG and LPS, produce activation of toll-like receptors (TLR) resulting in activation of innate immunity. In addition, endogenous 'alarmins' and chaperone proteins, including heat shock proteins (HSP), may activate adaptive and innate immunity and enhance the activity of vaccine therapies; their use is also being evaluated. Oncophage is an autologous HSP vaccine that reached Phase III trials in melanoma and renal cell cancer but the data were inconsistent.
- What is the optimal time to start vaccine therapies, how frequently should they be administered and at what intervals?

Immunostimulatory cytokines. Typically, immunostimulatory cytokines are used as adjuvants to augment the response to other immunotherapies, although some have been approved in Europe and the USA as standalone therapies (Table 3.4). IL-12 activates both innate (natural killer [NK] cells) and adaptive (cytotoxic T lymphocytes) immunities and has also been evaluated preclinically and in early phase clinical trials; however, results to date have been disappointing.[24]

TABLE 3.4

Immunostimulatory cytokines approved as cancer immunotherapies in Europe and/or the USA[12]

Cytokine	Indications
IL-2 (aldesleukin, Proleukin®)	Metastatic melanoma, renal cell carcinoma
IFN-α2b (Intron A®)	Melanoma, hairy cell leukemia, AIDS-related Kaposi's sarcoma, follicular lymphoma, cervical intraepithelial neoplasms
IFN-α2a (Roferon A®)	Hairy cell leukemia, chronic-phase Philadelphia chromosome-positive chronic myeloid leukemia (within 1 year of diagnosis)

AIDS, acquired immunodeficiency syndrome; IFN, interferon; IL, interleukin.

Cytokine antibodies and targeted agents. Pro-inflammatory cytokines have a role in the development of malignancy and regulation of the immune response to malignancy. IL-6 in particular plays a critical role in the differentiation of dendritic cells and of B cells into plasma cells, leading to production of antibodies. It is also important in regulating T helper cell function. In cancer, IL-6 is also important in:

- differentiation of myeloid-derived suppressor cells (MDSCs)
- regulation of self-renewal of cancer stem cells
- inhibition of apoptosis, thereby promoting tumor growth and progression
- enhancing angiogenesis
- the development of cancer cachexia syndrome.[25]

IL-6 signaling occurs through binding to the IL-6 receptor in conjunction with gp130 protein and activation of the JAK/STAT signaling pathway (janus kinase/signal transducer and activator of transcription). Antibodies to IL-6 have been successfully used in inflammatory conditions such as rheumatoid arthritis (RA), and tocilizumab is registered with the FDA for the treatment of adult and juvenile forms of RA. Therapeutic antibodies to IL-6 have also been trialed in cancer patients, including studies in the management of cancer cachexia syndrome.

Other cancer therapies target the JAK/STAT signaling pathway. However, despite encouraging results from a Phase II trial of the JAK 1 and 2 inhibitor ruxolitinib in patients with pretreated pancreatic cancer and elevated C-reactive protein concentrations,[26] two Phase III trials failed to improve outcomes.[27] There are also preliminary studies under way of antibodies targeting colony-stimulating factor receptors in order to influence dendritic cell and myeloid cell function in malignancy.

Immunomodulatory monoclonal antibodies. In contrast to the mAb therapies described on pages 38–9, immunomodulatory mAbs act by altering the function of various components of the immune system, thereby eliciting a new immune response or restoring an existing response. Such mAbs act in several ways:

- immune checkpoint blockade, including agents acting via the PD-1 receptor (e.g. pembrolizumab, nivolumab, atezolizumab) or CTLA-4 (e.g. ipilimumab) pathways

- activation of co-stimulatory receptors on the surface of immune effector cells, such as tumor necrosis factor (TNF) receptor superfamily member 4 (OX40)
- neutralization of immunosuppressive factors produced in the tumor microenvironment, such as transforming growth factor (TGF)-β.

Of these, immune checkpoint inhibitors are currently the only agents approved for clinical use in the EU and USA, largely based on clinical benefit shown in randomized Phase II or III clinical trials. Their clinical development and applications are detailed in the next chapter. Currently licensed products are listed in Table 3.5.

Inhibitors of immunosuppressant metabolism. Indoleamine 2,3-dioxygenase (IDO) catalyzes the first, rate-limiting, step in the metabolic pathway converting the essential amino acid tryptophan into kynurenine. IDO has a strong immunosuppressant effect,

TABLE 3.5

Immune checkpoint inhibitors approved in the EU and/or USA*

Agent	Target	Tumor type
Ipilimumab (Yervoy®)	CTLA-4	Melanoma
Pembrolizumab (Keytruda®)	PD-1	Melanoma, lung cancer, head and neck cancer, gastric cancer, Hodgkin's lymphoma, MSI-high solid tumors
Nivolumab (Opdivo®)	PD-1	Melanoma, lung cancer, kidney cancer, bladder cancer, colorectal cancer, Hodgkin's lymphoma
Atezolizumab (Tecentriq®)	PD-L1	Lung cancer, bladder cancer
Avelumab (Bavencio®)	PD-L1	Bladder cancer, Merkel cell cancer
Durvalumab (Imfinzi®)	PD-L1	Bladder cancer

*At the time of publication. Specific approved indications are detailed in Table 4.1. CTLA-4, cytotoxic T lymphocyte-associated protein 4; MSI-high, microsatellite instability-high; PD-1, programmed cell death-1 receptor; PD-L1, PD-1 ligand.

probably because of depletion of tryptophan in T cells, and has been implicated in the development of immune tolerance in cancer.

A number of small-molecule inhibitors of IDO have been investigated in clinical trials, and promising results have been obtained from a Phase II trial of a combination of an IDO inhibitor with the checkpoint inhibitor pembrolizumab in patients with advanced melanoma.[28] Further development in clinical trials is warranted.

Pattern recognition receptor (PRR) agonists are a class of proteins that recognize a variety of danger signals, including microbe-associated molecular patterns (MAMPs), such as bacterial LPS, and damage-associated molecular patterns (DAMPs), such as mitochondrial DNA. Examples of PRRs include toll-like receptors (TLRs) and nucleotide-binding oligomerization domain-containing (NOD)-like receptors (NLRs). PRRs play essential roles in the immune response to pathogens and in the reactivation of anticancer immune responses following chemotherapy, radiotherapy or immunotherapy.

A number of PRR agonists have been approved for use in cancer patients, including:
- BCG
- monophosphoryl lipid A, an LPS derivative used in the Cervarix® vaccine against HPV
- imiquimod, a trigger of TLR7 signaling that is used in the treatment of superficial basal cell carcinoma.

BCG is a live attenuated form of mycobacterium bovis that was introduced in 1921 as a vaccine against tuberculosis, and is still used for this purpose; it is the most widely used vaccine in the world. Several different strains of BCG are used worldwide and it is unclear which is the most effective. Use of BCG in the first 6 months of life halves mortality, presumably by increasing resistance to sepsis.

The anticancer effects of BCG result from the recruitment and activation of immune cells, including CD4+ T cells, which eliminate cancer cells that have internalized BCG. Administration of BCG also increases the number of monocytes and increases both pro- and anti-inflammatory cytokine production, as well as increasing production of interferon (IFN)-γ in unstimulated cells. It is used in cancer treatment as an intravesical adjuvant therapy to prevent recurrence of localized (non-muscle-invasive) bladder cancer.

Serious adverse events are uncommon (fewer than 8% of patients require treatment cessation for toxicity), although bladder irritation, malaise and fevers are common. Dose reduction and anti-inflammatory medications are usually effective in the management of significant side effects.[29]

Inducers of immunogenic cell death. Some forms of chemo- or radiotherapy can stimulate malignant cells to express DAMPs that bind to APCs, triggering a cancer-specific immune response via a process known as immunogenic cell death (ICD). Chemotherapy agents that have been shown to induce ICD include doxorubicin and related anthracyclines, bleomycin, oxaliplatin, cyclophosphamide and bortezomib.

Assessing the benefits and risks of immunotherapy in cancer

Assessment of the benefits and risks of cancer immunotherapies can be challenging, as the criteria used for conventional therapies cannot generally be extrapolated to immunotherapies.

Assessing efficacy. A key issue in immuno-oncology is that patients may show a survival benefit in the absence of an objective response as defined by conventional RECIST (Response Evaluation Criteria in Solid Tumors) criteria. Response to immunotherapies may vary markedly between patients: while some patients may show an initial response or stable disease, in others the response may be delayed because of the need to restore T-cell responses – a process that requires the interaction of numerous other immune cells. Indeed, in some patients, there is an initial phase of pseudoprogression during which the tumor appears to enlarge due to infiltration of newly reactivated T cells and subsequent inflammation.

For these reasons, a set of immune-related response criteria (irRC) have been proposed (Table 3.6), relating to four patterns of response:
- shrinkage of baseline lesions similar to that observed with conventional chemotherapy or targeted agents, without development of new lesions
- durable stable disease, which may be followed by a slow, steady decline in tumor burden in some patients
- response after an initial increase in tumor burden
- response in the presence of new lesions.

TABLE 3.6

Immune-related response criteria, compared with conventional RECIST criteria[30]

Response	irRC	RECIST
Complete response (CR)	Disappearance of all lesions in two consecutive observations ≥ 4 weeks apart	Disappearance of all target lesions; any pathological lymph nodes (whether target or non-target) must have reduction in short axis to < 10 mm
		Disappearance of all non-target lesions and normalization of tumor marker level; all lymph nodes must be non-pathological (< 10 mm short axis)
Partial response (PR)	≥ 50% decrease in tumor burden versus baseline in two observations ≥ 4 weeks apart	≥ 30% decrease in the sum of diameters of target lesions, taking as reference the baseline sum diameters
Stable disease (SD)	50% decrease in tumor burden versus baseline cannot be established, nor 25% increase versus nadir	Neither sufficient shrinkage to qualify for PR nor sufficient increase to qualify for PD, taking as reference the smallest sum diameters while on study
		Persistence of ≥ 1 non-target lesion(s) and/or maintenance of tumor marker level above the normal limits
Progressive disease (PD)	≥ 25% increase in tumor burden versus nadir (at any single time point) in two consecutive observations ≥ 4 weeks apart	≥ 20% increase in the sum of diameters of target lesions, taking as reference the smallest sum on study (including the baseline sum if that is the smallest on study); the sum must also demonstrate an absolute increase of ≥ 5 mm
		Unequivocal progression of existing non-target lesions
		The appearance of one or more new lesions is also considered progression*

(CONTINUED)

TABLE 3.6 (CONTINUED)

Immune-related response criteria, compared with conventional RECIST criteria[30]

Response category	irRC	RECIST
Non-index lesions (non-measurable or over allowed number)	Contribute to defining immune-related complete response (complete disappearance required)	Changes contribute to defining best overall response of CR or PR and SD or PD
New measurable lesions (≥ 5 × 5 mm)	Incorporated in tumor burden	Always represent progressive disease
New non-measurable lesions (≤ 5 × 5 mm, bone metastases, effusions)	Do not define progression (but preclude immune-related complete response)	Always represent progressive disease

*Non-CR/non-PD is preferred over SD when assessing non-target lesion disease.
irRC, immune-related response criteria; RECIST, Response Evaluation Criteria in Solid Tumors.

Assessing safety and tolerability. Some immunotherapies, notably checkpoint inhibitors, are associated with immune-related adverse events such as fatigue, diarrhea, nausea and altered liver or kidney function (Figure 3.4). Many of these resemble the adverse events often seen with conventional chemotherapy but have different etiologies: while adverse events with conventional chemotherapy usually reflect cytotoxic effects on healthy tissue, adverse events with immunotherapies typically reflect actions on the immune system. For example, diarrhea associated with immunotherapy may be due to a reaction to gut-associated or self-antigens.

Such adverse events require careful management, because although most are mild or moderate in severity, failure to recognize them as

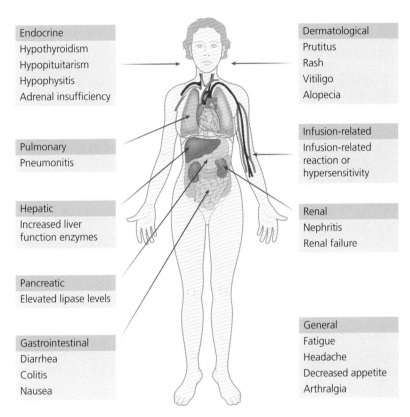

Endocrine
Hypothyroidism
Hypopituitarism
Hypophysitis
Adrenal insufficiency

Pulmonary
Pneumonitis

Hepatic
Increased liver
function enzymes

Pancreatic
Elevated lipase levels

Gastrointestinal
Diarrhea
Colitis
Nausea

Dermatological
Prutitus
Rash
Vitiligo
Alopecia

Infusion-related
Infusion-related
reaction or
hypersensitivity

Renal
Nephritis
Renal failure

General
Fatigue
Headache
Decreased appetite
Arthralgia

Figure 3.4 Immune-related adverse events. Adapted from Kreamer 2014.[8]

immune related could lead to suboptimal management, with potentially serious or life-threatening consequences. For example, if untreated, diarrhea from immune-related colitis may become self-perpetuating, potentially leading to gut perforation.

Patient education about such adverse events is essential: patients should be warned not to ignore 'slight' or 'mild' symptoms, but to seek medical advice as soon as possible. A multidisciplinary approach, involving oncologists, organ specialists and intensive care physicians, is essential for patients with severe immune-related adverse events.

In rare cases, cytokine release syndrome (CRS) may occur as a result of inflammatory cytokine release following administration of mAbs or BiTEs, or in patients undergoing CAR-T therapy. This syndrome is

TABLE 3.7

Symptoms of cytokine release syndrome

Systemic	Organ-related	Laboratory findings
• Fever	• Oliguria	• Hypokalemia
• Chills	• Bronchospasm	• Increased urea
• Headache	• Dyspnea	• Decreased GFR
• Asthenia	• Hypotension	• Altered blood counts, coagulation tests or both
• Myalgia	• Tachycardia	
• Arthralgia	• Arrhythmia	
• Back or abdominal pain	• Confusion	• Elevated CRP, procalcitonin or both
	• Erythema	
	• Urticarial reactions	
	• Pruritus	

CRP, C-reactive protein; GFR, glomerular filtration rate.

characterized by diverse systemic and organ-related symptoms that occur during or immediately after infusion of the antibody (Table 3.7). CRS can usually be managed symptomatically but in severe cases it may be necessary to use a mAb directed against IL-6, such as tocilizumab, to reverse the inflammatory process.

Combining immuno-oncology drugs and other treatments
As experience with immunotherapies in oncology accumulates, attention is turning to the possibility of combining immunotherapy with other treatment modalities.

Combining different immunotherapies. Combinations of immunotherapies acting on different immune pathways offers the potential for additive or synergistic antitumor activity. Studies in patients with melanoma receiving a combination of the CTLA-4 inhibitor ipilimumab and the PD-1 inhibitor nivolumab suggest that the combination is significantly more effective than ipilimumab alone;[31] on the basis of these findings, the FDA has approved this combination for the treatment of *BRAF* wild-type advanced melanoma. Combinations of CTLA-4 inhibitors and PD-1/PD-L1 inhibitors are being investigated in other cancers, including non-small-cell lung cancer (NSCLC) and renal cell carcinoma.

Combining immunotherapy with targeted therapies. Combinations of checkpoint inhibitors and targeted inhibitors of the BRAF and MEK oncoproteins are being investigated in patients with metastatic melanoma and other solid tumors. A Phase I trial with ipilimumab and the BRAF inhibitor vemurafenib was halted prematurely because of severe hepatotoxicity,[32] but this has not been seen with other BRAF inhibitors. Preclinical data suggest that a combination of PD-1 blockade with anti-BRAF therapy may be beneficial in advanced melanoma; this approach is being investigated.

Combining immunotherapy with chemotherapy. As described above, certain forms of chemotherapy can sensitize tumors to immunotherapy by promoting ICD. Similarly, some other chemotherapies, such as cisplatin, can enhance the efficacy of T cell-based immunotherapies by sensitizing the malignant cells to T cell-induced death rather than by ICD.

Clinical trials in patients with advanced melanoma have found that the addition of dacarbazine to ipilimumab increased response rates and produced a slight increase in overall survival, compared with dacarbazine alone, but these benefits were achieved at the cost of an increased rate of severe (grade 3/4) immune-related adverse events.[33]

A randomized Phase II trial of carboplatin and pemetrexed with and without pembrolizumab showed improved response rates (55% versus 29%, $p = 0.0032$) and progression-free survival (13 versus 8.9 months, $p = 0.0205$) with the combination in patients with untreated advanced NSCLC.[34] This provided the basis for accelerated FDA approval of the chemo-immunotherapy combination for patients with untreated advanced NSCLC. The confirmatory Phase III randomized trial is ongoing.

Combining immunotherapy with radiotherapy. Radiotherapy can modulate local and systemic immune responses, possibly through ICD, increased uptake of tumor antigens by dendritic cells and by enhancing CD8+ T-cell responses. Although this effect is not sufficient to overcome immune tolerance in cancer cells, the combination of radiotherapy with immunotherapy may be beneficial. To date, however, clinical trials of this strategy have shown that such combinations are less toxic than combinations of immune checkpoint inhibitors with targeted therapies, but local and distant (abscopal) anti-tumor responses are limited.

Key points – how cancer immunotherapy works

- The term immunotherapy encompasses a variety of approaches, targeting diverse immunologic targets.
- The potential sensitivity of a given cancer to immunotherapy depends on the immunogenicity of the tumor, which is related to the somatic mutation rate within tumor cells.
  - The highest mutation rates are seen in cancers of the skin, lung, bladder and stomach, rendering these tumor types more sensitive to immunotherapy.
- Immunotherapies are conventionally classified as passive or active, depending on their ability to activate an immune response against tumor cells.
  - Passive immunotherapies include tumor-targeting monoclonal antibodies, adoptive cell transfer and oncolytic viruses.
  - Active immunotherapies include dendritic cell-based therapies, vaccines, immunomodulatory monoclonal antibodies (immune checkpoint inhibitors) and pattern recognition receptor agonists.
- Efficacy criteria used for conventional cancer therapies cannot readily be extrapolated to immunotherapies.
  - Survival may be increased in the absence of an objective response as assessed by conventional criteria, and hence immune-related response criteria are required.
- Immune-related adverse events are generally due to autoimmune inflammation through uncontrolled T-cell activation.
  - Such events should be treated promptly to prevent potentially harmful escalation: patient education is essential in this respect.

References

1 Kamta J, Chaar M, Ande A et al. Advancing cancer therapy with present and emerging immuno-oncology approaches. *Front Oncol* 2017;7:64.

2 Messerschmidt JL, Prendergast GC, Messerschmidt GL. How cancers escape immune destruction and mechanisms of action for the new significantly active immune therapies: helping nonimmunologists decipher recent advances. *Oncologist* 2016;21:233–43.

3 Ehrlich P. Über den jetzigen Stand der Karzinomforschung. *Ned Tijdschr Geneeskd* 1909;5:273–90.

4 Thomas L. Discussion. In: *Cellular and Humoral Aspects of the Hypersensitive States*. Lawrence HS, ed. New York: Hoeber-Harper, 1959:529–32.

5 Burnet M. Cancer – a biological approach. *Br Med J* 1957;1:779–86.

6 Dunn GP, Bruce AT, Ikeda H, Schreiber RD. Cancer immunoediting: from immunosurveillance to tumor escape. *Nat Immunol* 2002;3:991–8.

7 Leach DR, Krummel MF, Allison JP. Enhancement of antitumor immunity by CTLA-4 blockade. *Science* 1996;271:1734–6.

8 Kreamer KM. Immune checkpoint blockade: a new paradigm in treating advanced cancer. *J Adv Pract Oncol* 2014;5:418–31.

9 Wang J, Yuan R, Song W et al. PD-1, PD-L1 (B7-H1) and tumor-site immune modulation therapy: the historical perspective. *J Hematol Oncol* 2017;10:34.

10 Rajasagi M, Shukla SA, Fritsch EF et al. Systematic identification of personal tumor-specific neoantigens in chronic lymphocytic leukemia. *Blood* 2014;124:453–62.

11 Lawrence MS, Stojanov P, Polak P et al. Mutational heterogeneity in cancer and the search for new cancer-associated genes. *Nature* 2013;499:214–18.

12 Galluzzi L, Vacchelli E, Bravo-San Pedro JM et al. Classification of current anticancer immunotherapies. *Oncotarget* 2014;5:12472–508.

13 Heslop HE, Slobod KS, Pule MA et al. Long-term outcome of EBV-specific T-cell infusions to prevent or treat EBV-related lymphoproliferative disease in transplant recipients. *Blood* 2010;115:925–35.

14 Porter DL, Levine BL, Kalos M et al. Chimeric antigen receptor-modified T cells in chronic lymphoid leukemia. *N Engl J Med* 2011;365: 725–33.

15 Brentjens RJ, Davila ML, Riviere I et al. CD19-targeted T cells rapidly induce molecular remissions in adults with chemotherapy-refractory acute lymphoblastic leukemia. *Sci Transl Med* 2013;5:177ra38.

16 Grupp SA, Laetsch TW, Buechner J et al. Analysis of a global registration trial of the efficacy and safety of CTL019 in pediatric and young adults with relapsed/refractory acute lymphoblastic leukemia. *Blood* 2016;128:Abstract 221.

17 Andtbacka RH, Kaufman HL, Collichio F et al. Talimogene laherparepvec improves durable response rate in patients with advanced melanoma. *J Clin Oncol* 2015;33:2780–8.

18 Chang MH, Chen CJ, Lai MS et al. Universal hepatitis B vaccination in Taiwan and the incidence of hepatocellular carcinoma in children. Taiwan Childhood Hepatoma Study Group. *N Engl J Med* 1997;336:1855–9.

19 Jit M, Brisson M, Portnoy A, Hutubessy R. Cost-effectiveness of female human papillomavirus vaccination in 179 countries: a PRIME modelling study. *Lancet Glob Health* 2014;2:e406–14.

20 Sabado RL, Balan S, Bhardwaj N. Dendritic cell-based immunotherapy. *Cell Res* 2017;27:74–95.

21 Kantoff PW, Higano CS, Shore ND et al. Sipuleucel-T immunotherapy for castration-resistant prostate cancer. *N Engl J Med* 2010;363:411–22.

22 Vansteenkiste JF, Cho BC, Vanakesa T et al. Efficacy of the MAGE-A3 cancer immunotherapeutic as adjuvant therapy in patients with resected MAGE-A3-positive non-small-cell lung cancer (MAGRIT): a randomised, double-blind, placebo-controlled, phase 3 trial. *Lancet Oncol* 2016;17:822–35.

23 Weller M, Butowski N, Tran DD et al. Rindopepimut with temozolomide for patients with newly diagnosed, EGFRvIII-expressing glioblastoma (ACT IV): a randomised, double-blind, international phase 3 trial. *Lancet Oncol* 2017;18:1373–85.

24 Portielje JE, Lamers CH, Kruit WH et al. Repeated administrations of interleukin (IL)-12 are associated with persistently elevated plasma levels of IL-10 and declining IFN-gamma, tumor necrosis factor-alpha, IL-6, and IL-8 responses. *Clin Cancer Res* 2003;9:76–83.

25 Yao X, Huang J, Zhong H et al. Targeting interleukin-6 in inflammatory autoimmune diseases and cancers. *Pharmacol Ther* 2014;141:125–39.

26 Hurwitz HI, Uppal N, Wagner SA et al. Randomized, double-blind, Phase II study of ruxolitinib or placebo in combination with capecitabine in patients with metastatic pancreatic cancer for whom therapy with gemcitabine has failed. *J Clin Oncol* 2015;33:4039–47.

27 Hurwitz H, Van Cutsem E, Bendell JC et al. Two randomized, placebo-controlled phase 3 studies of ruxolitinib (Rux) + capecitabine (C) in patients (pts) with advanced/metastatic pancreatic cancer (mPC) after failure/intolerance of first-line chemotherapy: JANUS 1 (J1) and JANUS 2 (J2). *J Clin Oncol* 2017;35(Suppl 4):343.

28 Zakharia Y, McWilliams R, Shaheen M et al. Interim analysis of the Phase 2 clinical trial of the IDO pathway inhibitor indoximod in combination with pembrolizumab for patients with advanced melanoma. Presented at the 107th Annual Meeting of the American Association for Cancer Research (AACR), 1–5 April 2017; Washington, DC. Abstract CT117.

29 Martínez-Piñeiro JA, Jiménez León J, Martínez-Piñeiro L Jr et al. Bacillus Calmette-Guerin versus doxorubicin versus thiotepa: a randomized prospective study in 202 patients with superficial bladder cancer. *J Urol* 1990;143:502.

30 Wolchok JD, Hoos A, O'Day S et al. Guidelines for the evaluation of immune therapy activity in solid tumors: immune-related response criteria. *Clin Cancer Res* 2009;15:7412–20.

31 Wolchok JD, Chiarion-Sileni V, Gonzalez R et al. Overall survival with combined nivolumab and ipilimumab in advanced melanoma. *N Engl J Med* 2017;377:1345–56.

32 Ribas A, Hodi FS, Callahan M et al. Hepatotoxicity with combination of vemurafenib and ipilimumab. *N Engl J Med* 2013;368:1365–6.

33 Robert C, Thomas L, Bondarenko I et al. Ipilimumab plus dacarbazine for previously untreated metastatic melanoma. *N Engl J Med* 2011;364:2517–26.

34 Langer CJ, Gadgeel SM, Borghaei H et al. Carboplatin and pemetrexed with or without pembrolizumab for advanced, non-squamous non-small-cell lung cancer: a randomised, phase 2 cohort of the open-label KEYNOTE-021 study. *Lancet Oncol* 2016;17: 1497–508.

Further reading

Baruch EN, Berg AL, Besser MJ et al. Adoptive T cell therapy: An overview of obstacles and opportunities. *Cancer* 2017;123:2154–62.

Chen DS, Mellman I. Oncology meets immunology: the cancer-immunity cycle. *Immunity* 2013;39: 1–10.

Fountzilas C, Patel S, Mahalingam D. Review: oncolytic virotherapy, updates and future directions. *Oncotarget* 31 May 2017. doi: 10.18632/oncotarget.18309 [Epub ahead of print].

Kroschinsky F, Stölzel F, von Bonin S et al. New drugs, new toxicities: severe side effects of modern targeted and immunotherapy of cancer and their management. *Crit Care* 2017;21:89.

Medina PJ, Adams VR. PD-1 pathway inhibitors: immuno-oncology agents for restoring antitumor immune responses. *Pharmacotherapy* 2016;36:317–34.

Swart M, Verbrugge I, Beltman JB. Combination approaches with immune-checkpoint blockade in cancer therapy. *Front Oncol* 2016;6:233.

4 Clinical use of immune checkpoint inhibitors

Recent years have seen unparalleled advances in the clinical development of immune checkpoint inhibitors targeting the programmed cell death-1 receptor (PD-1) and its ligand PD-L1 and cytotoxic T lymphocyte-associated protein 4 (CTLA-4). The rationale for targeting these immune checkpoints, and the clinical experience with these agents, are discussed here.

Immune checkpoint molecules

Immune checkpoint molecules are cell surface receptors that are expressed on activated T cells and other immune cells, which normally serve a co-inhibitory role in keeping the adaptive immune system in check to prevent autoimmune diseases.

CTLA-4 is the first immune checkpoint found to be expressed by immune cells, especially T regulatory cells (T_{reg}) and activated T cells that have been acutely exposed to antigens. When bound to CD80 (B7-1) and CD86 (B7-2) on antigen-presenting cells (APCs), CTLA-4 acts as an off switch to down-regulate the immune response (Figure 4.1).

PD-1 is another immune checkpoint expressed by activated T cells, B cells and macrophages. PD-1 signaling may inhibit T-cell activation by binding to either one of two ligands, PD-L1 (B7-H1) or PD-L2 (B7-DC). As described in Chapter 2, the PD-L1/2 ligands may be expressed on tumor cells and immune cells in the tumor microenvironment, thus inhibiting effector T cells (T_{eff}) and preventing an adequate immune response on cancer (see Figure 4.1).

Checkpoint inhibition. CTLA-4, PD-1 and PD-L1 therefore represent attractive therapeutic targets where checkpoint inhibition by monoclonal antibodies (mAbs) helps activate T-cell function to uncover and attack cancer cells. The analogy of releasing the brakes to accelerate a fast car has been widely used to explain this mechanism of action.

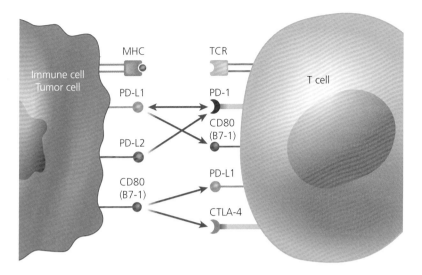

Figure 4.1 Checkpoint molecules are cell surface receptors that are expressed on activated T cells and other immune cells. Upon T-cell activation, programmed cell death 1 (PD-1) and CTLA-4 receptors are expressed on T cells. When the PD-1 and/or CTLA-4 receptors are coupled to the programmed cell death ligand 1 or ligand 2 (PD-L1/2) or B7-1 (CD80)/B7-2 (CD86), respectively on the tumor cell, the normal immune response is inhibited, preventing an attack on the tumor cell. Therefore, monoclonal antibody (mAb)-mediated blockade of these pathways prevents inhibition of T-cell function and enhances anti-tumor immunity.

Antibodies against PD-1/PD-L1

This is one of the most prolific areas of drug development at present, and many pharmaceutical companies have a PD-1 or PD-L1 mAb in late-stage clinical development. Those approved by the US Food and Drug Administration (FDA) are summarized in Table 4.1. As can be seen, the registration status of the various mAbs differs; pembrolizumab and nivolumab have the widest indications at present. Pembrolizumab and nivolumab are mAbs against PD-1, on the surface of T cells, while avelumab, durvalumab and atezolizumab block tumor-based PD-L1. While there have been modest differences in clinical outcomes in different tumors, there is currently little evidence of significant differences between these agents in terms of their clinical activity and toxicity profiles.

TABLE 4.1

Mechanism of action and indications of FDA-approved PD-1/PD-L1 monoclonal antibodies*

Nivolumab (Opdivo®)/BMS
PD-1 antibody – human IgG4

Indications:
- Unresectable or metastatic melanoma
- In combination with ipilumimab for unresectable or metastatic melanoma
- Advanced renal cell carcinoma after prior anti-angiogenic therapy
- Locally advanced or metastatic urothelial cancers after progression on platinum-containing chemotherapy
- Metastatic NSCLC – second line
- Recurrent or metastatic HNSCC – second line
- MSI-high CRC after progression on chemotherapy
- Classic Hodgkin's lymphoma after autologous transplantation and brentuximab

Pembrolizumab (Keytruda®)/MSD
PD-1 antibody – human IgG4

Indications:
- Initial treatment of patients with unresectable or metastatic melanoma
- Unresectable or metastatic melanoma
- Recurrent or metastatic HNSCC – second line
- Locally advanced or metastatic urothelial cancers after progression on platinum-containing chemotherapy
- MSI-high CRC, after progression on chemotherapy
- MSI-high advanced solid tumors
- Advanced NSCLC with PD-L1 ≥ 50% – first line
- In combination with carboplatin and pemetrexed for metastatic non-squamous NSCLC – first line
- Metastatic NSCLC with PD-L1 expression – second line
- Recurrent or metastatic HNSCC – second line
- Hodgkin's lymphoma – refractory or ≥ 3 lines of chemotherapy
- Gastric cancer with PD-L1 expression – third line

(CONTINUED)

TABLE 4.1 (CONTINUED)

Mechanism of action and indications of FDA-approved PD-1/PD-L1 antibodies*

Avelumab (Bavencio®)/EMD Serono
PD-L1 blocking human IgG1 lambda

Indications:
- Locally advanced or metastatic urothelial cancers after progression on platinum-containing chemotherapy
- Metastatic Merkel cell cancer

Durvalumab (Imfinzi®)/AstraZeneca:
PD-L1 blocking human IgG1 kappa

Indications:
- Locally advanced or metastatic urothelial cancers after progression on platinum-containing chemotherapy

Atezolizumab (Tecentriq®)/Genentech
PD-L1 blocking human IgG1

Indications:
- Locally advanced or metastatic urothelial cancers after progression on platinum-containing chemotherapy
- Metastatic NSCLC – second line

*At the time of publication.
CRC, colorectal cancer; FDA, Food and Drug Administration; HNSCC, head and neck squamous cell carcinoma; Ig, immunoglobulin; MSI, microsatellite instability; NSCLC, non-small-cell lung cancer; PD-1, programmed cell death receptor-1; PD-L1, programmed cell death receptor ligand.

Antibodies targeting CTLA-4

Ipilimumab (Yevoy®, BMS) and tremelimumab (AstraZeneca) are antibodies targeting CTLA-4 that have reached Phase III trials, but to date only ipilimumab has been approved by the FDA as adjuvant therapy, in patients with melanoma. Approval was based on a positive Phase III randomized trial in patients with resected stage III melanoma, which showed improved recurrence-free and overall survival compared with placebo.[1]

Clinical activity of PD-1/PD-L1 and CTLA-4 targeted antibodies

Table 4.2 summarizes the results of Phase III studies with checkpoint inhibitors at the time of writing.

TABLE 4.2

Examples of completed Phase III clinical trials with checkpoint inhibitors

Tumor type (trial name)	Stage/other feature(s)	Drug
Melanoma (CA184-024)[2,3]	Previously treated	Ipilimumab, 10 mg/kg + dacarbazine, 850 mg/m² vs placebo + dacarbazine
Melanoma (CA184-002)[4]	Previously treated, HLA-A*0201 positive, stage 3 or 4	3:1:1 Ipilimumab, 3 mg/kg + gp100 vs ipilimumab, 3 mg/kg vs gp100
Melanoma (KeyNote 006)[5,6]	≤ 1 prior therapy for advanced melanoma	1:1:1 Pembrolizumab (P), 10 mg/kg q 2/52 vs 3/52 vs ipilimumab (I), 3 mg/kg 4 doses
Melanoma (CheckMate 067)[7,8]	First line	Nivolumab vs ipilimumab vs combination
Melanoma (CheckMate 066)[9]	Previously untreated, but without *BRAF* mutation	Nivolumab, 3 mg/kg + placebo q 2/52 vs dacarbazine, 1000 mg/m² + placebo
Melanoma (CA184-169)[10]	First line for IO	Ipilimumab, 10 mg/kg vs 3 mg/kg
Melanoma (CheckMate 037)[11]	Progression on ipilimumab	Nivolumab vs CT
Melanoma[12]	First line	Tremelimumab, 15 mg/kg vs CT
Melanoma (EORTC 18071)[1]	Adjuvant	Ipilimumab vs placebo
Urothelial carcinoma (Keynote 045)[13]	Second-line post-platinum failure	Pembrolizumab vs CT
Renal cell carcinoma (CheckMate 025)[14]	Second line	Nivolumab, 3 mg/kg vs everolimus, 10 mg daily
NSCLC (CheckMate 026)[15]	First line in PD-L1 ≥ 5%	Nivolumab, 3 mg/kg vs platinum-based CT

RR (%)	Overall survival (median unless otherwise stated)
33.2 vs 30.2 NS	11.2 vs 9.1 months, $p < 0.001$ 5-year survival: 18.2% vs 8.8%
5.7 vs 11 vs 1.5	10.1 vs 10.0 vs 6.4 months, $p = 0.003$ 12-month survival: 43.6 vs 45.6 vs 25.3% 24-month survival: 21.6 vs 23.5 vs 13.7%
33.7 (P2/52) vs 32.9 (P3/52) vs 11.9 (I)	NR (P arms) vs 16 (I) months 2-year survival: 55% (P2/52) vs 55% (P3/52) vs 43% (I)
43.7 (N) vs 19 (I) vs 57.6 (N + I)	37.6 (N) vs 19.9 (I) vs NR (N + I) months
40 vs 13.9, $p < 0.001$	1-year survival: 72.9% vs 42.1% 2-year survival: 46.3% vs 26.7% Median OS not reached for patients on nivolumab
15 (10) vs 12 (3)	15.7 (10) vs 11.5 (3) months, $p = 0.04$
27 vs 10	16 vs 14 months (NS)
10.7 vs 9.8	12.6 vs 10.7 months (NS)
–	5-year survival: 65.4% vs 54.4% RFS: 40.8% vs 30.3%
21 vs 11, $p = 0.0001$	10.3 vs 7.4 months, $p = 0.002$
25 vs 5, $p < 0.001$	25 vs 19.6 months, $p \leq 0.0148$
26 vs 33	14.4 vs 13.2 months (NS)

TABLE 4.2 (CONTINUED)

Examples of completed Phase III clinical trials with checkpoint inhibitors

Tumor type (trial name)	Stage/other feature(s)	Drug
NSCLC (KeyNote 024)[16]	First line in PD-L1 ≥ 50%	Pembrolizumab, 200 mg q 3/52 vs CT
Squamous NSCLC (CheckMate 017)[17]	Second-line after CT	Nivolumab, 3 mg/kg vs docetaxel, 75 mg/m² q 3/52
Non-squamous NSCLC (CheckMate 057)[18]	Second-line after CT	Nivolumab, 3 mg/kg vs docetaxel, 75 mg/m² q 3/52
NSCLC (KeyNote 010)[19]	Second-line after CT; PD-L1 ≥ 1%	Pembrolizumab, 2 mg/kg (P2) vs 10 mg/kg (P10), both q 3/52 vs docetaxel (D), 75 mg/m² q 3/52
NSCLC (OAK)[20]	Second/third-line after CT	Atezolizumab, 1200 mg vs docetaxel,75 mg/m² q 3/52
SCLC (CA184-156)[21]	First-line, extensive stage	EP + ipilimumab, 10 mg/kg vs EP + placebo q 3/52
Head and neck SCC (CheckMate 141)[22]	Second-line after platinum CT (< 6 months)	Nivolumab vs systemic therapy (methotrexate, docetaxel or cetuximab) 2:1
Prostate (CA184-043)[23]	Post-docetaxel after 8 Gy single-fraction RT in CRPC with ≥ 1 bony metastasis	Ipilimumab, 10 mg/kg or placebo q 3/52
Prostate (CA184-095)[24]	CRPC with asymptomatic or minimal symptoms	Ipilimumab, 10 mg/kg vs placebo 2:1

CRPC, castration-resistant prostate cancer; CT, chemotherapy; EP, etoposide platinum chemotherapy; gp, glycoprotein; HRQoL, health-related quality of life; NR, not reached; NS, not significant; NSCLC, non-small-cell lung cancer; PD-1, programmed cell death receptor-1; PD-L1, PD-1 receptor ligand; RFS, relapse-free survival; RR, response rate; RT, radiotherapy; SCC, squamous cell carcinoma; SCLC, small cell lung cancer.

RR (%)	Overall survival (median unless otherwise stated)
44.8 vs 27.8, p not given	6-month survival: 80.2% vs 72.4%, $p < 0.005$ Median survival: NR
20 vs 9, $p = 0.008$	9.2 vs 6.0 months, $p < 0.001$
19 vs 12, $p = 0.02$	12.2 vs 9.4 months, $p = 0.002$
18 (P2) vs 18 (P10) vs 9 (D) – higher in ≥ 50% PD-L1 expression	10.4 (P2) vs 12.7 (P10) vs 8.5 (D) months, $p = 0.0008$ (P2 vs D) and $p < 0.0001$ (P10 vs D)
–	13.8 vs 9.6 months, $p = 0.0003$
62 vs 62	11 (I) vs 10.9 (placebo) (NS)
13.3 vs 5.8	7.5 vs 5.1 months, $p = 0.01$ Improved HRQoL
–	11.2 (I) vs 10.0 (placebo) (NS)
	28.7 (I) vs 29.7 (placebo) (NS)

Many more trials are under way or recently completed, including studies in other tumor types, and metastatic, adjuvant and neoadjuvant treatment settings, and studies of combinations of checkpoint inhibitors with systemic therapies, including chemotherapy, other targeted agents and radiotherapy.

Malignant melanoma. Data are most mature for the treatment of malignant melanoma. The experience gained in this setting indicates that traditional endpoints, such as response rates and median progression-free and overall survival, do not reflect the true value of treatment with checkpoint inhibitors: more important is the percentage of patients surviving long term without active malignancy, the so called 'tail of the curve'. The PD-1 targeting antibodies are more active than the CTLA-4 targeting agents, but combinations of the two increase long-term survival rates, albeit with increased toxicity.[7] Responses have also been achieved in patients with brain metastases.[25]

Lung cancer. Single-agent PD-1/PD-L1 mAbs have consistently shown improvements in median survival of approximately 3 months compared with chemotherapy in patients receiving second-line treatment for non-small-cell lung cancer (NSCLC).[26] Response rates are higher in patients whose tumors have higher expression of PD-L1, although responses also occur in patients with low or no expression.

Studies comparing nivolumab or pembrolizumab with chemotherapy as first-line therapy have shown conflicting results, probably because of differences in patient selection between trials. Compared with chemotherapy, pembrolizumab produced higher response rates (45% versus 28%), a 4-month improvement in median progression-free survival (10 versus 6 months) and better overall survival at 6 months (80% versus 72%) in patients with 50% or more tumor expression of PD-L1.[16] In contrast, nivolumab provided no progression-free or overall survival advantage over standard chemotherapy in patients with 5% or more tumor PD-L1 expression.[15] As in melanoma, responses have been seen in patients with brain metastases.[27]

Urological malignancies. Improved response and survival rates, compared with standard therapies, have been seen in randomized trials of pembrolizumab and nivolumab as second-line treatment for urothelial and renal cell cancers, respectively.[13,14] By contrast, no such improvements have been seen with ipilimumab in men with castration-resistant prostate cancer.[23,24]

Gastrointestinal malignancies. Checkpoint inhibitors have not proved effective in patients with pancreatic cancer or microsatellite stable colorectal cancers. However, 26–50% of patients with high microsatellite instability (MSI-high) colorectal cancer responded to checkpoint inhibitors in Phase II trials, but with evidence of protracted responses; Phase III trials are under way.[28]

There have also been encouraging results in hepatocellular and esophagogastric cancers, and further confirmatory studies are under way.

Head and neck cancer. Nivolumab has been shown to produce modest improvements in response rates and overall survival, compared with standard chemotherapy, in patients with head and neck squamous cell carcinoma that has relapsed after platinum-based chemotherapy.[22] Pembrolizumab has demonstrated durable responses in a Phase II multi-cohort trial, and a Phase III trial is ongoing.

Lymphoma. Both nivolumab and pembrolizumab have shown impressive high and durable response rates in patients with both Hodgkin's disease and non-Hodgkin's lymphoma. However, further studies will be required to determine the optimal use of these agents in these diseases.

Merkel cell cancer is an uncommon and aggressive skin cancer that may be associated with Merkel cell polyomavirus, and also occurs in the elderly after significant sun exposure. A large Phase II study of avelumab in 88 patients with stage IV Merkel cell cancer that had progressed after chemotherapy showed a response rate of 32%, including eight complete responses. At a median follow-up of 10 months, 82% of responses were ongoing.[29] Activity has also been demonstrated with other agents.

Mesothelioma. High levels of PD-L1 have been associated with non-epithelioid histology and reduced survival in patients with mesothelioma. A Phase II study of pembrolizumab demonstrated a response rate of 24% in 25 mesothelioma patients with disease progression after chemotherapy.[30] Other studies with PD-1 or PD-L1 antibodies and CTLA-4-targeted drugs are under way or recently completed.

Other cancers. There is a strong rationale for using immunotherapies in other tumors, including glioblastoma and triple-negative breast cancer, but mature clinical data are awaited.

Toxicities from checkpoint inhibitors

The biggest limitation to the use of checkpoint inhibitors has been toxicity, even though tolerability is generally superior to chemotherapy. Immune-related adverse events usually result from autoimmune inflammation of various organs due to over-activation of T cells. Severe toxicities can lead to interruption and/or cessation of therapy, substantial morbidity and occasional mortality. Sometimes expensive therapies may be needed to effectively manage adverse effects that do not respond to steroids. At present, there are no effective predictors of toxicities. Nevertheless, a number of general statements can be made regarding the toxicities of checkpoint inhibitors.

- Patients in clinical trials have been highly selected for performance status and good organ function and thus toxicities may be worse in non-trial patient populations. Patients with pre-existing autoimmune toxicities have been excluded from trials of immunotherapies and thus toxicities may be greater in this group.
- Adverse events can affect any organ system but gastrointestinal, skin, hepatic and endocrine toxicities are most common.
- Toxicities are more common with combinations of a PD-1/PD-L1 inhibitor with a CTLA-4 targeted agent than with monotherapies.[31,32] It has not been possible to deliver the same doses of combination therapies used in melanoma to lung cancer patients.
- Grade 3/4 toxicities have been reported in fewer than 3% of patients treated with PD-1/PD-L1 inhibitors;[33] 9% treated with ipilimumab monotherapy, but 19% of patients who received combination therapy.

- Diarrhea of all grades occurs in 11–19% (grade 3/4 in 0–3%) of patients receiving PD-1 mAbs, and up to one-third of ipilimumab-treated patients (grade 3/4 in 3–6%). However, with combination therapy, diarrhea occurs in up to 44% of patients (grade 3/4 9%). Diarrhea typically appears at a median of 7 weeks with ipilimumab and nivolumab, compared with 6 months with pembrolizumab. Colitis (diarrhea, pain and bleeding/mucous) may develop in a small percentage of patients receiving PD-L1 mAbs, but occurs in 8–12% of both ipilimumab-treated (grade 3/4 in 3–6%) and combination-treated patients (grade 3/4 in 9%). Occasionally, patients experience gastrointestinal perforation or severe colitis requiring colectomy.
- Abnormalities in liver function tests, predominantly alanine transaminase/aspartate transaminase (ALT/AST) elevations, occur in 1–6% of patients treated with PD-L1 mAbs (grade 3/4 in 1–3%) and 1–7% of ipilimumab-treated patients (grade 3/4 in 0–2%), compared with 30% of patients receiving combination therapy (grade 3/4 in 19%). Liver dysfunction typically occurs 6–12 weeks after starting treatment.
- Skin toxicities, including pruritus and rash, occur in 14–22% (grade 3/4 in < 1%) of PD-1 mAb-treated patients, 15–35% of ipilimumab-treated patients (grade 3/4 in 1–2%) and 28–33% of patients receiving combination therapy (grade 3/4 2–3%). Vitiligo occurs in 5–11%, 2–4% and 7%, respectively. Skin toxicities are more common in patients with melanoma than in patients with other tumor types.
- Alterations in endocrine function are common. For example, evidence of hypothyroidism occurs in 4–10% of patients treated with PD-1 mAbs, 2–4% of ipilimumab-treated patients and 15% of combination-treated patients, although it is rarely severe. Similarly, hyperthyroidism occurs in 2–7%, 1–2% and 10%, respectively, but again is rarely severe. Fewer than 2% of patients receiving single agents have pituitary function abnormalities, compared with 8% of those who receive combination treatment.
- Pneumonitis is more common in patients with lung cancer than in those with melanoma. With the PD-1 mAbs, up to 5% of patients with lung cancer experience pneumonitis, which may be grade 3/4 in up to 2%. The incidence appears to be greater in patients who

have received significant thoracic radiotherapy. PD-1 mAbs appear to be associated with higher rates of pneumonitis than PD-L1 mAbs.[34]

- Rheumatological toxicities, including arthralgias and myalgias, occur in 6–12% of patients, but are rarely severe or treatment limiting.
- Fatigue occurs in 15–34% of patients receiving single-agent therapy and 35% of those receiving combination treatment, among whom it may be severe in up to 4%.
- Neurological toxicities are uncommon (< 1%), but may be severe and include Guillain–Barre syndrome.
- The timing of the onset of toxicities may differ even between members of the same class of agent (Figure 4.2).

Management of toxicities

Patients and staff should be educated about the types of toxicity associated with immunotherapies, and patients should be provided with a card indicating that they are receiving a particular treatment. Emergency department staff should be offered educational sessions. Expert nurses with knowledge of toxicities and their management should be employed to monitor patients' symptoms and provide education and advice about toxicity management. Toxicity grading systems should be understood. Local experts in the management of gastrointestinal, skin, endocrine, pulmonary and neurological toxicities should be identified and included in the multidisciplinary team.

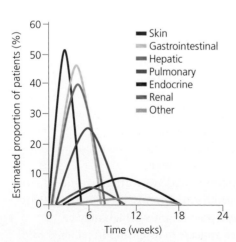

Figure 4.2 Incidences, onset and resolution of immune-mediated toxicities of the PD-1 checkpoint inhibitors nivolumab and pembrolizumab (pooled data from pivotal trials reported by the European Medicines Agency). Reproduced with permission from Eigentler et al. 2016.[33]

For diarrhea and colitis, treatment should be interrupted and steroids (methylprednisolone, 2 mg/kg/day intravenously) should be initiated if toxicity is greater than grade 2 or if there is abdominal pain or more than six bowel motions per day. Infliximab should be initiated if there is no improvement after 48–72 hours and colitis is confirmed on endoscopy. Permanent discontinuation of immunotherapy should be considered for patients with toxicity greater than grade 3 (Figure 4.3).[35]

For liver dysfunction, treatment should be interrupted in cases of grade 2 toxicity or greater, and steroids (prednisone, 1 mg/kg orally, or

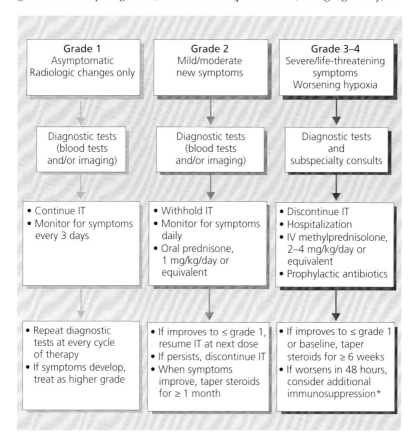

Figure 4.3. Management of immune-related adverse events. *Infliximab, cyclophosphamide, mycophenolate mofetil. CT, computed tomography; IT, immunotherapy; IV, intravenous. Adapted from Naidoo et al. 2015.[35]

methylprednisolone, 2 mg/kg/day intravenously) initiated for grade 2 toxicity or greater. If there is no response within the first few days, a trial of mycophenylate, 500–1000 mg twice daily, should be considered.

Pneumonitis should be observed if asymptomatic. In symptomatic patients, treatment should be interrupted and steroids initiated as above for liver dysfunction. Other immunosuppressive agents, such as mycophenylate, antithymocyte globulin or infliximab, can be added if the patient's condition does not improve.

Key points – clinical use of immune checkpoint inhibitors

- Immune checkpoints are cell surface receptors that are expressed on activated T cells and other immune cells, which normally serve a co-inhibitory role in keeping the adaptive immune system in check to prevent autoimmune diseases.
- Immune checkpoints may be inhibited by monoclonal antibodies, resulting in T-cell activation and an immune response against cancer. This is analogous to releasing the brakes to accelerate a fast car.
- Immune checkpoint inhibitors against CTLA-4, PD-1 and PD-L1 have produced durable tumor shrinkage and prolonged survival in patients with a variety of solid tumors.
- Immune checkpoint inhibitors have been approved by the US Food and Drug Administration for use in patients with melanoma, lung cancers, head and neck cancers, bladder cancers, kidney cancers, colorectal cancers, MSI-high solid tumors, Merkel cell cancers and Hodgkin's lymphoma. These include ipilimumab (CTLA-4 mAb), nivolumab, pembrolizumab (PD-1 mAbs), atezolizumab, avelumab and durvalumab (PD-L1 mAbs).
- Clinical trials are ongoing for additional indications, as well as various combination therapies.
- Immune-related adverse events are due to autoimmune inflammation resulting from overactivation of T cells; they include colitis, dermatitis, hepatitis, thyroiditis and pneumonitis.

References

1 Eggermont AM, Chiarion-Sileni V, Grob JJ, et al. Prolonged survival in stage III melanoma with ipilimumab adjuvant therapy. *N Engl J Med* 2016; 375:1845–55.

2 Robert C, Thomas L, Bondarenko I et al. Ipilimumab plus dacarbazine for previously untreated metastatic melanoma. *N Engl J Med* 2011;364:2517–26.

3 Maio M, Grob JJ, Aamdal S et al. Five-year survival rates for treatment-naive patients with advanced melanoma who received ipilimumab plus dacarbazine in a phase III trial. *J Clin Oncol* 2015;33:1191–6.

4 Hodi FS, O'day SJ, Mcdermott DF et al. Improved survival with ipilimumab in patients with metastatic melanoma. *N Engl J Med* 2010;363:711–23.

5 Robert C, Schachter J, Long GV et al. Pembrolizumab versus ipilimumab in advanced melanoma. *N Engl J Med* 2015;372:2521–32.

6 Schachter J, Ribas A, Long GV et al. Pembrolizumab versus ipilimumab for advanced melanoma: final overall survival results of a multicentre, randomised, open-label phase 3 study (KEYNOTE-006). *Lancet* 2017;Aug 16. pii:S0140-6736(17)31601-X.

7 Larkin J, Chiarion-Sileni V, Gonzalez R et al. Combined nivolumab and ipilimumab or monotherapy in untreated melanoma. *N Engl J Med* 2015;373:23–34.

8 Wolchok JD, Chiarion-Sileni V, Gonzalez R et al. Overall survival with combined nivolumab and ipilimumab in advanced melanoma. *N Engl J Med* 2017;377:1345–56.

9 Robert C, Long GV, Brady B et al. Nivolumab in previously untreated melanoma without *BRAF* mutation. *N Engl J Med* 2015;372:320–30.

10 Ascierto PA, Del Vecchio M, Robert C et al. Ipilimumab 10 mg/kg versus ipilimumab 3 mg/kg in patients with unresectable or metastatic melanoma: a randomised, double-blind, multicentre, phase 3 trial. *Lancet Oncol* 2017;18:611–22.

11 Larkin J, Minor D, D'angelo S et al. Overall survival in patients with advanced melanoma who received nivolumab versus investigator's choice chemotherapy in CheckMate 037: a randomized, controlled, open-label phase III trial. *J Clin Oncol* 2017;JCO2016718023 [Epub ahead of print].

12 Ribas A, Kefford R, Marshall MA et al. Phase III randomized clinical trial comparing tremelimumab with standard-of-care chemotherapy in patients with advanced melanoma. *J Clin Oncol* 2013;31:616–22.

13 Bellmunt J, De Wit R, Vaughn DJ et al. Pembrolizumab as second-line therapy for advanced urothelial carcinoma. *N Engl J Med* 2017;376:1015–26.

14 Motzer RJ, Escudier B, Mcdermott DF et al. Nivolumab versus everolimus in advanced renal-cell carcinoma. *N Engl J Med* 2015;373:1803–13.

15 Carbone DP, Reck M, Paz-Ares L et al. First-line nivolumab in stage IV or recurrent non-small-cell lung cancer. *N Engl J Med* 2017;376: 2415–26.

16 Reck M, Rodríguez-Abreu D, Robinson AG et al. Pembrolizumab versus chemotherapy for PD-L1-positive non-small-cell lung cancer. *N Engl J Med* 2016;375:1823–33.

17 Brahmer J, Reckamp KL, Baas P et al. Nivolumab versus docetaxel in advanced squamous-cell non-small-cell lung cancer. *N Engl J Med* 2015;373:123–35.

18 Borghaei H, Paz-Ares L, Horn L et al. Nivolumab versus docetaxel in advanced nonsquamous non-small-cell lung cancer. *N Engl J Med* 2015;373:1627–39.

19 Herbst RS, Baas P, Kim DW et al. Pembrolizumab versus docetaxel for previously treated, PD-L1-positive, advanced non-small-cell lung cancer (KEYNOTE-010): a randomised controlled trial. *Lancet* 2016;387:1540–50.

20 Rittmeyer A, Barlesi F, Waterkamp D et al. Atezolizumab versus docetaxel in patients with previously treated non-small-cell lung cancer (OAK): a phase 3, open-label, multicentre randomised controlled trial. *Lancet* 2017;389:255–65.

21 Reck M, Luft A, Szczesna A et al. Phase III randomized trial of ipilimumab plus etoposide and platinum versus placebo plus etoposide and platinum in extensive-stage small-cell lung cancer. *J Clin Oncol* 2016;JCO676601 [Epub ahead of print].

22 Ferris RL, Blumenschein G Jr., Fayette J et al. Nivolumab for recurrent squamous-cell carcinoma of the head and neck. *N Engl J Med* 2016;375:1856–67.

23 Kwon ED, Drake CG, Scher HI et al. Ipilimumab versus placebo after radiotherapy in patients with metastatic castration-resistant prostate cancer that had progressed after docetaxel chemotherapy (CA184-043): a multicentre, randomised, double-blind, phase 3 trial. *Lancet Oncol* 2014;15:700–12.

24 Beer TM, Kwon ED, Drake CG et al. Randomized, double-blind, phase III trial of ipilimumab versus placebo in asymptomatic or minimally symptomatic patients with metastatic chemotherapy-naive castration-resistant prostate cancer. *J Clin Oncol* 2017;35:40–7.

25 Margolin K, Ernstoff MS, Hamid O et al. Ipilimumab in patients with melanoma and brain metastases: an open-label, phase 2 trial. *Lancet Oncol* 2012;13:459–65.

26 Malhotra J, Jabbour SK, Aisner J. Current state of immunotherapy for non-small cell lung cancer. *Transl Lung Cancer Res* 2017;6:196–211.

27 Goldberg SB, Gettinger SN, Mahajan A et al. Pembrolizumab for patients with melanoma or non-small-cell lung cancer and untreated brain metastases: early analysis of a non-randomised, open-label, phase 2 trial. *Lancet Oncol* 2016;17:976–83.

28 Le DT, Uram JN, Wang H et al. PD-1 blockade in tumors with mismatch-repair deficiency. *N Engl J Med* 2015;372:2509–20.

29 Kaufman HL, Russell J, Hamid O et al. Avelumab in patients with chemotherapy-refractory metastatic Merkel cell carcinoma: a multicentre, single-group, open-label, phase 2 trial. *Lancet Oncol* 2016;17:1374–85.

30 Alley EW, Lopez J, Santoro A et al. Clinical safety and activity of pembrolizumab in patients with malignant pleural mesothelioma (KEYNOTE-028): preliminary results from a non-randomised, open-label, phase 1b trial. *Lancet Oncol* 2017;18:623–30.

31 Hassel JC, Heinzerling L, Aberle J et al. Combined immune checkpoint blockade (anti-PD-1/anti-CTLA-4): evaluation and management of adverse drug reactions. *Cancer Treat Rev* 2017;57:36–49.

32 De Velasco G, Je Y, Bosse D et al. Comprehensive meta-analysis of key immune-related adverse events from CTLA-4 and PD-1/PD-L1 inhibitors in cancer patients. *Cancer Immunol Res* 2017;5:312–18.

33 Eigentler TK, Hassel JC, Berking C et al. Diagnosis, monitoring and management of immune-related adverse drug reactions of anti-PD-1 antibody therapy. *Cancer Treat Rev* 2016;45:7–18.

34 Khunger M, Rakshit S, Pasupuleti V et al. Incidence of pneumonitis with use of programmed death 1 and programmed death-ligand 1 inhibitors in non-small cell lung cancer: a systematic review and meta-analysis of trials. *Chest* 2017;152:271–81.

35 Naidoo J, Page DB, Li BT, Connell LC et al. Toxicities of the anti-PD-1 and anti-PD-L1 immune checkpoint antibodies. *Ann Oncol* 2015;26:2375–91.

Further reading

Kamta J, Chaar M, Ande A et al. Advancing cancer therapy with present and emerging immuno-oncology approaches. *Front Oncol* 2017;7:64.

Kroschinsky F, Stölzel F, von Bonin S et al. New drugs, new toxicities: severe side effects of modern targeted and immunotherapy of cancer and their management. *Crit Care* 2017;21:89.

5　The future of immuno-oncology

Immunotherapy has already become an essential component of standard treatment for patients with advanced cancer. The most advanced treatments are the immune checkpoint inhibiting monoclonal antibodies (mAbs) that target the programmed cell death 1 (PD-1)/programmed cell death ligand 1 (PD-L1) axis and cytotoxic T lymphocyte-associated 4 protein (CTLA-4). Vaccine therapies have shown some promise, and are especially appealing because of a lack of serious toxicities, but interest in these has been somewhat overshadowed by the success of the mAbs.

Where we are today

In advanced malignant melanoma, which was incurable in the era of chemotherapy, we are now seeing durable long-term remission in many patients with the use of combination immunotherapies, including in patients with brain metastases. In patients with lung cancer, we are seeing excellent responses and survival in more than 20% of patients, and certain products have also been approved for use after failure of initial therapy in head and neck squamous cell carcinoma, urothelial cancer and renal cell carcinoma. Moreover, there also seems to be substantial clinical activity in some uncommon malignancies, such as Merkel cell cancer, mesothelioma and relapsed lymphoma. The US Food and Drug Administration (FDA) has also recently approved PD-1/PD-L1 inhibitors for the treatment of microsatellite unstable tumors following exciting clinical activity, especially in high microsatellite instability (MSI-high) colorectal cancer.

Despite these encouraging developments, the outcomes with immunotherapies have been less encouraging in other common malignancies such as microsatellite stable colorectal cancer and pancreatic cancer. As a result, combinations with other targeted immunotherapies or chemotherapy are now being extensively investigated. It is too early to gauge the place of immunotherapy in some other common malignancies, because pivotal clinical trials are still ongoing. Clearly, a number of important issues around the use of cancer immunotherapies remain to be resolved. Some of the most important of these are highlighted here.

Developments in immuno-oncology have created justifiable excitement. However, the optimal use of this multitude of therapies requires ongoing clinical evaluation, guided by appropriate preclinical models and translational science.

Who will/won't benefit from treatment

Despite the clinical breakthroughs described above, at present most patients do not respond to immunotherapy, even for an approved indication. In clinical practice, the lack of precision therapy is compounded by a range of unpredictable and often serious immune-related adverse events that require careful management.

The lack of reliable predictive biomarkers of efficacy or toxicity is perhaps the major current issue around the use of immunotherapies. At present, the best predictor of benefit from immune checkpoint inhibitors is mutational burden,[1,2] but this cannot be routinely assessed, particularly in a serial fashion in patients receiving treatment. Liquid biopsies with plasma-circulating tumor DNA may provide a non-invasive tool to explore this, but much more research is required in this area.[3]

While there is some correlation between levels of PD-L1 expression and response and survival in lung cancer, these relationships lack sensitivity and specificity, and this situation is further complicated by the availability of multiple separate testing platforms, with variable correlation between them. In other tumor types, especially melanoma, there appears to be no such correlation.

A further issue with the measurement of PD-L1 levels in patients with lung cancer has been the requirement for a core biopsy. This is difficult to do via an endoscopic approach, and patients are usually required to have a more invasive radiological biopsy that requires greater expertise and carries an increased risk of complications such as bleeding and pneumothorax. Levels of immune proteins in peripheral venous blood samples are currently being evaluated as potential biomarkers of response.

Preliminary data suggest that elevated systemic inflammatory markers may identify patients who are less likely to benefit from immunotherapy in the advanced disease setting. Further clarification of this relationship, and determination of the optimal systemic inflammatory marker, may improve patient selection and provide options for future combination therapies. Such analyses are likely to be less useful in earlier stages of disease when inflammatory markers are less frequently elevated.[4]

Optimal combinations of immunotherapies with other anti-cancer treatments

Combination therapies with PD-1/PD-L1 mAbs and CTLA-4-targeted drugs provide greater responses and survival than monotherapies in patients with melanoma, albeit with significantly greater autoimmune toxicities. However, to date, patients with lung cancer have not tolerated the same doses as those given to patients with melanoma. These combinations are now being explored in other cancer types.

Studies are under way with combinations of established immunotherapies and new agents that target other immune regulatory molecules, including activating antibodies that target agonistic immune receptors and inhibitory antibodies that target inhibitory immune receptors. It is hoped that these combinations will be efficacious in malignancies that are currently resistant to immunotherapies.

Optimal use of cancer vaccines and oncolytic viruses will involve:
- upregulation of dendritic cell, CD8+ T cell and natural killer (NK) cell functions
- inhibition of immunosuppressive pathways regulated by myeloid suppressor cells and cytokines such as interleukin (IL)-6.

This will require combination therapy with checkpoint inhibitors in addition to janus kinase/signal transducer and activator of transcription (JAK/STAT) inhibitors and other modulators of acute inflammation, including IL-6 antibodies. Clearly, the optimal use of vaccines and other immunotherapies in combination with standard systemic therapies, radiotherapy and surgery needs to be established.

Immunotherapies plus systemic therapies. Early data from patients with lung cancer suggest that added benefit can be obtained from the combination of chemotherapy and immunotherapy. For example, in the Keynote 021 study, which involved patients with stage IIIB/IV non-squamous non-small-cell lung cancer (NSCLC), the response rate among patients receiving carboplatin, pemetrexed and pembrolizumab was 55% (95% CI 42–68), compared with 29% (95% CI 18–41%, $p = 0.0016$) for patients receiving chemotherapy alone. Median progression-free survival was 13 months (95% CI 8.3 to not reached) for the pembrolizumab arm, compared with 8.9 months (95% CI 4.4–10.3) for the chemotherapy arm (HR 0.53 [95% CI 0.31–0.91] $p = 0.010$). Rates of grade 3 or greater toxicities were similar in the two arms.[5] The data from the Phase III trial Keynote-189 are awaited.

Multiple trials are under way to determine whether there is benefit in adding an immunotherapeutic agent – be it a checkpoint inhibitor, or a vaccine or their combination – to chemotherapy, targeted agents or other systemically delivered anti-cancer therapies. It will be exciting to see if concurrent or prior use of other systemic therapies might increase mutational burden, and thereby improve the response to immunotherapies.

There are also data showing that certain types of chemotherapy, including the anthracyclines, oxaliplatin and cyclophosphamide, induce immunogenic cell death (ICD), a process that results in the release of damage-associated molecular patterns (DAMPs), such as the membrane-bound calreticulin and high-mobility group box 1 (HMGB1) proteins from the nucleus. These proteins cause binding and activation of antigen-presenting cells (APCs) and release of proinflammatory cytokines that further activate the immune system (Figure 5.1). A similar process may occur with radiotherapy (see below). Therapeutic exploitation of ICD in conjunction with checkpoint inhibitors is a logical next step in combination therapies.

Immunotherapies plus radiation. Radiotherapy is widely used to treat patients with malignancy in a number of settings, including curative, adjuvant and palliative treatment. As well as external beam radiotherapy and brachytherapy, radiation is also involved in the form of therapeutic isotopes and selective internal radiation delivery. Radiation can induce ICD, creating the potential for synergy with immunotherapies, especially the immune checkpoint inhibitors. ICD may be responsible in whole or part for the 'abscopal effect', in which, in addition to cell death at an irradiated site, an anti-tumor effect also occurs at distant sites of disease that have not been irradiated.[6]

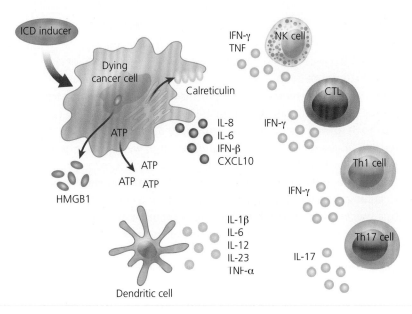

Figure 5.1 Induction of immunogenic cell death (ICD) in cancer cells. ICD inducers trigger the release of damage-associated molecular patterns (DAMPs) and inflammatory cytokines, which signal to dendritic cells and natural killer (NK) cells that in turn release effector cytokines. Consequently, T cells differentiate into cytotoxic lymphocytes (CTLs) or T_h1/T_h17 cells, releasing additional effector cytokines. IFN, interferon; IL, interleukin; TNF, tumor necrosis factor. Adapted from Showalter A et al. 2017.[8]

Preclinical evidence suggests synergy between radiotherapy and antibodies to CTLA-4 and PD-L1, which is thought to be because ionizing radiation causes a local vaccine-like effect.

Clinical trials are under way to determine the optimal dose and scheduling of radiotherapy to combine with immunotherapies. It appears that standard scheduling of radiotherapy provides more favorable immune interaction than hypofractionated schedules.[7,8] Also, preliminary data show that the presence of higher densities of CD45RO+ tumor-infiltrating lymphocytes (TILs) is associated with better prognosis in patients with rectal cancer, while higher densities of CD3+ and CD8+ TILs and lower fractions of regulatory T cells are associated with better response to radiotherapy.[9] Monitoring of these associations will be useful in ongoing combination studies.

Optimal timing of immunotherapy interventions

To date, therapeutic antibodies that target immune checkpoint inhibitors, and immune therapies in general, have predominantly been used in the advanced disease setting, initially in patients who have received prior therapy. The future of immuno-oncology will be to define whether these agents might be more effective when given in the postoperative adjuvant setting, or even in the neoadjuvant setting prior to definitive surgery. In preclinical murine models of triple-negative breast cancer, neoadjuvant immunotherapy involving depletion of regulatory T cells reduced rates of metastatic disease and increased numbers of long-term survivors compared with the same treatment given in a postsurgical adjuvant fashion.[10] Similarly, the use of anti-PD-1 therapies in the neoadjuvant setting produced longer survival than adjuvant treatment, albeit without long-term survivors. However, this was improved when an anti-CD137 antibody was added to the anti-PD-1 agent in the neoadjuvant, but not adjuvant, setting. This effect was shown to be dependent on the presence of interferon-γ and tumor-specific circulating CD8+ cells.

A number of studies of neoadjuvant therapy in various tumor settings are under way. Some Phase III studies of adjuvant immunotherapy completed in patients with resected melanoma have demonstrated improvements in disease-free survival but long-term survival data are awaited.[11] Similarly, a randomized trial of adjuvant durvalumab versus placebo showed significantly improved progression-free survival in patients with stage III non-small-cell lung cancer after chemoradiotherapy.[12]

Optimal duration of immunotherapies

The optimal duration of treatment with immunotherapies is unknown. The duration of therapy in clinical trials is highly arbitrary: for example, the duration of ipilimumab treatment in patients with melanoma was 4 doses over 3 months in the metastatic setting, and up to 3 years in the adjuvant setting.[11,13] For PD-1 mAbs, some patients are treated indefinitely and others for up to 2 years. It is currently unclear whether long-term responders need ongoing costly infusions of these immunotherapies at the same dosing intervals.

Prediction and management of immunotherapy toxicities

Toxicity is the greatest limitation to the use of combinations of immunotherapies. Overall toxicities are less than with chemotherapy, but a small percentage of patients experience severe and life-threatening toxicities such as colitis, pneumonitis, hepatitis and neurological impairment, including Guillain–Barre syndrome. The toxicities are more severe with the combination of a PD-1/PD-L1 targeted drug and a CTLA-4-inhibiting mAb, and are greater in some tumor types (e.g. lung compared with melanoma).

An ability to predict or completely control toxicities would greatly enhance the use of combination immunotherapies. Similarly, it would be helpful to know how to use these agents safely in patients with pre-existing autoimmune diseases, transplant recipients and those with intercurrent infection.

Precision immunotherapy

Immuno-oncology has made incredible advances in recent years. In order to harness the immune system for enhanced anti-tumor response and deliver optimal immunotherapy to every patient, predictive biomarkers and novel combination treatment strategies are urgently needed. In the future, the one size fits all model will become obsolete, and precision immunotherapy will be tailored to each individual to radically improve their outcomes.

Key points – the future of immuno-oncology

- Predictive biomarkers are urgently needed to direct precision immunotherapy.
- Tumor mutation burden is a promising predictor of response to immune checkpoint inhibitors but requires further study, including the use of non-invasive tools such as plasma-circulating tumor DNA analysis.
- Predictive biomarkers for immune-related toxicity are also needed.
- Combinations of immune checkpoint inhibitors with targeted therapy, chemotherapy or radiotherapy are being explored to see whether responses may be augmented.

References

1 Snyder A, Makarov V, Merghoub T et al. Genetic basis for clinical response to CTLA-4 blockade in melanoma. *N Engl J Med* 2014;371:2189–99.

2 Rizvi NA, Hellmann MD, Snyder A et al. Cancer immunology. Mutational landscape determines sensitivity to PD-1 blockade in non-small cell lung cancer. *Science* 2015;348:124–8.

3 Gandara DR, Kowanetz M, Mok TSK et al. Blood-based biomarkers for cancer immunotherapy: tumor mutational burden in blood (bTMB) is associated with improved atezolizumab (atezo) efficacy in 2L+ NSCLC (POPLAR and OAK). *Ann Oncol* 2017;28(suppl_5): v460–96.

4 Diakos CI, Charles KA, McMillan DC et al. Cancer-related inflammation and treatment effectiveness. *Lancet Oncol* 2014;15:e493–503.

5 Langer CJ, Gadgeel SM, Borghaei H et al. Carboplatin and pemetrexed with or without pembrolizumab for advanced, non-squamous non-small-cell lung cancer: a randomised, phase 2 cohort of the open-label KEYNOTE-021 study. *Lancet Oncol* 2016;17:1497–508.

6 Postow MA, Callahan MK, Barker CA et al. Immunologic correlates of the abscopal effect in a patient with melanoma. *N Engl J Med* 2012;366:925–31.

7 Bernier J. Immuno-oncology: allying forces of radio- and immuno-therapy to enhance cancer cell killing. *Crit Rev Oncol Hematol* 2016;108:97–108.

8 Showalter A, Limaye A, Oyer JL et al. Cytokines in immunogenic cell death: applications for cancer immunotherapy. *Cytokine* 2017;97:123–32.

9 Wang L, Zhai ZW, Ji DB et al. Prognostic value of CD45RO(+) tumor-infiltrating lymphocytes for locally advanced rectal cancer following 30 Gy/10f neoadjuvant radiotherapy. *Int J Colorectal Dis* 2015;30:753–60.

10 Liu J, Blake SJ, Yong MC et al. Improved efficacy of neoadjuvant compared to adjuvant immunotherapy to eradicate metastatic disease. *Cancer Discov* 2016;6:1382–99.

11 Eggermont AM, Chiarion-Sileni V, Grob JJ et al. Prolonged survival in stage III melanoma with ipilimumab adjuvant therapy. *N Engl J Med* 2016;375:1845–55.

12 Antonia SJ, Villegas A, Daniel D et al. Durvalumab after chemoradiotherapy in stage III non–small-cell lung cancer. *N Engl J Med* 2017;8 September [Epub ahead of print].

13 Hodi FS, O'Day SJ, McDermott DF et al. Improved survival with ipilimumab in patients with metastatic melanoma. *N Engl J Med* 2010;363:711–23.

Useful resources

UK

British Association for Cancer Research
www.bacr.org.uk

British Society for Immunology
Tel: +44 (0)20 3019 5901
BSI@immunology.org
www.immunology.org

USA

American Association for Cancer Research
Tel: +1 215 440 9300
aacr@aacr.org
www.aacr.org

American Society of Clinical Oncology
Tel: +1 571 483 1780
Toll-free: 1 888 651 3038
contactus@cancer.net
www.asco.org

Institute for Clinical Immuno-oncology
Tel: +1 301 984 9496
iclio@accc-cancer.org
www.accc-iclio.org

International

Association for Cancer Immunotherapy
office@cimt.eu
www.cimt.eu

Clinical Oncology Society of Australia
Tel: +61 (0)2 8063 4100
cosa@cancer.org.au
www.cosa.org.au

European Association for Cancer Research
Tel: +44 (0)115 951 5060
hello@eacr.org
www.eacr.org

European Society for Medical Oncology
Tel: +41 (0)91 973 19 00
www.esmo.org

Society for Immunotherapy of Cancer
Tel: +1 414-271-2456
info@sitcancer.org
www.sitcancer.org

FastTest

You've read the book ... now test yourself with key questions from the authors

- Go to the FastTest for this title *FREE* at fastfacts.com
- Approximate time **10 minutes**
- For best retention of the key issues, try taking the FastTest before and after reading

Index